So you want to
Live Younger
Longer?

Also by Dr Norman Swan

So You Think You Know What's Good for You?

Dr NORMAN SWAN

So you want to Live Younger Longer?

**The ultimate guide to longevity
from Australia's most trusted doctor**

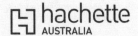

Published in Australia and New Zealand in 2022
by Hachette Australia
(an imprint of Hachette Australia Pty Limited)
Gadigal Country, Level 17, 207 Kent Street, Sydney, NSW 2000
www.hachette.com.au

Hachette Australia acknowledges and pays our respects to the past, present and future Traditional Owners and Custodians of Country throughout Australia and recognises the continuation of cultural, spiritual and educational practices of Aboriginal and Torres Strait Islander peoples. Our head office is located on the lands of the Gadigal people of the Eora Nation.

 A catalogue record for this work is available from the National Library of Australia

ISBN: 978 0 7336 4834 2 (paperback)

Cover design by Christabella Designs
Cover image courtesy of Getty Images
Author photo courtesy of Janie Barrett
Typeset in Minion Pro by Kirby Jones
Printed and bound in Australia by McPherson's Printing Group

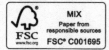

The paper this book is printed on is certified against the Forest Stewardship Council® Standards. McPherson's Printing Group holds FSC® chain of custody certification SA-COC-005379. FSC® promotes environmentally responsible, socially beneficial and economically viable management of the world's forests.

For Esther, Matilda and Nicholas.
I love you so much.

Contents

Introduction

Explanations exist; they have existed for all time; there is always a well-known solution to every human problem – neat, plausible, and wrong.
H.L. Mencken, 1920, *Prejudices: Second Series*

Dunno about you but I intend to live forever

Yep, I know it's ridiculous but I've had a fear of dying since I was eight years old. Funnily enough, on the couple of occasions when I've acutely confronted the imminent possibility of dying, I was too preoccupied to feel fear. No, the fear is more about going silently in the night. While I've made programs on advanced care planning – even done it myself – and on palliative care (which, by the way, can actually extend life), when my time comes, if I have the choice I'll rail against the inevitable and not give up easily.

Death stuck its nose into my life at the age of eight. Jack was my only uncle. He was young, good looking and unusually for a Glaswegian, especially a Jewish one, was very physically active outdoors. He got sick in his mid-20s with what I much later discovered was leukaemia. It was in the days before sophisticated chemo and bone marrow transplants and he died at 28. But here's the thing. I wasn't told for weeks. We just stopped going to the hospital and he wasn't mentioned in conversation. Ever again. My mother and grandmother were clearly distraught but that wasn't new. They had been for a long time while Jackie was ill. When eventually I was told, my mother admonished me not to say anything about it and never to say his name again because it would be too upsetting for her and my grandparents. And so never was his memory honoured or Jack's name spoken again in our family – to the extent that we didn't follow Jewish tradition of naming a child after a recently deceased loved one. When my youngest brother was born, he was only given Jack's middle name, Phillip. As I write this, I'm surprising myself about how hard it is, even now all these years later, to tell the story. I'm not doing it in some pop-psychological fashion to dump my issues on you but more to give some context to why I'm resolute in pushing my fate out as far as possible.

My motivation? I want to know what happens next ... How will world affairs play out? How will my family evolve? Will my apartment become a waterfront thanks to global warming? What sort of world could it be without my oversized, narcissistic ego in it?

I suppose the first thing to say is that in a global context it's almost an indecent luxury to be thinking and writing about all the keeping young stuff – looking good, being fit, on the ball and out of the hands of the medical system. I grew up in the West of Scotland, where the life expectancy difference between the longest-lived (least deprived) area and the shortest-lived (most deprived) is currently 13 years for men and 10 years for women. I now live in a country where the life expectancy gap between the kind of suburb I live in (a well-off metro suburb) and the shortest-lived area (APY Lands in northwest South Australia) is 41 years. Forty-one. But the factors that predict a long and healthy life are the same in remote Aboriginal communities as in affluent suburbs. They're just so much more difficult to achieve structurally because the bottom line is that a fair society, identity, control and the ways we distribute wealth, knowledge and resources are the underpinnings of staying young as long as possible.

Despite my egoistical fear, my rebellion against the inevitable is not at any cost. I don't jump from one new shiny thing to another and there are a lot of shiny things out there flogging perpetual energy, thinness, high-definition muscles, a life without wrinkles and high octane brain function. My promise to you is not to point my finger at you or tell you what to do but sift the rubbish from the gold and let you make up your own mind.

While the Book of Life (see later) starts to get written during pregnancy, it's remarkable what can be done to stay younger longer at all ages.

My uncle Jack (I never did have any other uncles or aunts) would now be nearly 90 if he'd survived and I sometimes wonder how he'd have been in old age. If my mother and father were anything to go by, he might not have been in great shape. They did live into their 90s but did not age well. Years of smoking earlier in life, no daily physical activity and an appalling diet, which for most of their lives was a mix of the worst of Glaswegian and Jewish cuisine, played havoc with their health and the rapidity with which their bodies aged. Modern medicine, a bucket load of drugs each day and aged care support kept them going.

The goal of this book regardless of your age is to help you get to your 90s and beyond in the body and with the brain of someone much younger. As you'll discover, it needs a bit of work. So if you've picked up this book in the shop looking for an easy answer, don't buy it. Get one that promises something simple and unbelievable.

What is this staying young thing?

#youwish

Quick take: Many of us have a tendency to focus on the physical aspects of staying young, such as being lean and fit, careful about what we eat, what supplements we should take and how we look, and I will cover those. However, you can do all that and be disappointed because you may not solve why you feel older than you are. At each stage in life we tend to have an ideal age in mind. Young kids look at teenagers and wish they were them. Adolescents look at young adults and want to jump to that stage of life. At some point there's a flip and we either want to stay the age we are or have an ideal younger age in mind. Interestingly, that disappears in the elderly, who often reach a happy acceptance. The point I'm making is that a lot of this is about attitudes, feelings, stress and general physical health. You won't know you're living younger longer if you don't feel it.

What is this staying young thing? Well, the answer to this depends on when you start thinking about it. Let's assume that's common when the big birthdays with a 4, 5 or 6 in front of them approach. When the Big 4 looms, it doesn't do you any good to hear someone like me saying, 'Jeez, if only I could be 40 again,' when I can barely remember what happened yesterday much less years ago. And there's a buyer be wary warning here. I originally trained to be a paediatrician, so what do I know about grown-ups? Like many men, I must admit there has been the occasional person in my life who's seriously questioned the extent to which I have actually grown up. What I will say, though, is that while there's an enormous knowledge base on child development and the stages babies, young kids and adolescents go through, there's relatively little research about how adults develop once they've left the turbulence and fractiousness of adolescence (some say that's about the age of 27 for men). Studies which have followed groups of people since early adulthood have tended to focus on how illnesses develop rather than how you evolve as a person.

So let's make some assumptions at the get-go.

What you look for depends on your age, stage, your 'people' (i.e. who you feel you belong with), your gender identity, who you're responsible and care for, whether you feel financially and emotionally secure, and a long list of other factors. Once we're into adulthood, we tend to look back at earlier ages and wonder how we managed to stay up till 3 a.m. in bars having what we thought at the time were deep and meaningful conversations but of which we now can't recall a single one. Or we wistfully recall a vigour that we feel has been burnt off by caring for children, mortgage repayments and career anxiety.

There is a thing called 'felt age' – the age we feel we are, independent of how many years we actually have on the clock. Studies of both younger and older people show that you feel older on days when the stress is piling on or when you're feeling physically unwell. And to flip that, you feel younger when you don't feel put upon and are in good health. Older people also feel younger the more control they think they have over their lives. Many of us also have a sense of how young we'd *like* to be and while a lot of people are very happy being the age they are, the gap between your felt age and your ideal age widens on days when you're feeling low, stressed or experiencing physical symptoms. Often these factors are intertwined and feed off each other.

Bottom line here is that you can spend a fortune on plastic surgery, personal trainers and supplements, but they won't necessarily make you feel younger even though every last wrinkle has been paralysed by botox. Disappointment can haunt you. Good plastic surgeons know this and are careful to find out what their clients' expectations are. These surgeons know that hell hath no fury like an angry, disappointed, out-of-pocket patient.

You can't live longer younger unless you feel younger and the research suggests that our prime tasks include staying well, noticing what's chronically stressing you and whether you're able to do something about it, and if your mood is low and staying low, seeking help for it. Although, as you'll find out later, there are things you can do yourself to raise your mood.

The other side of this is that if you feel younger than you are, it's probably a good indication that you probably are younger than your age on the clock (chronological age).

The Book of Life

#genesarentdestiny

Short sermon: There are ten days in the Jewish calendar between New Year (Rosh Hashanah) and the Day of Atonement (the fast of Yom Kippur) which are driven by the belief that at the beginning of each year God writes your destiny in the Book of Life. She decides who's going to be around next Rosh Hashanah and who isn't. So you'd better repent and get your shit together to do better. The modern version is that a geneticist does that for you. The idea is that you need a long-lived mum, dad, pop or nan to live long yourself. For the first time in human history, that's far less true. But there are some things written into your genetic Book of Life and you'd better know them so they can be identified and counteracted (if possible). (See Get Out of Those Genes.)

I'm named after an uncle of my mother who died young and my middle name is from another relative of hers who also died young by today's standards. The common story in those days was that you retired and died a year or two later. Very few people in my family were in good shape. I do, however, have a photo of my paternal grandfather (who landed in Glasgow from Lithuania at the age of eight) looking very fit. Apparently he took up wrestling in his youth, presumably to help survive the Gorbals – a slum suburb where immigrants found their first homes. Didn't help much in the long term, though, because cigarettes killed him at the age of 67. As I mentioned, my own parents crept through to their 90s, mostly as triumphs of modern medicine. They never took a day's deliberate exercise in their lives and there wasn't much incidental activity either. So I'm not at all sure what my genes tell me about my own longevity because the generations before me had to survive adversity and very unhealthy lifestyles.

In the past few decades there's been a quiet revolution in the thinking about the genetics of longevity. It used to be thought that to live long and in good health you really needed to have parents who lived long and well, and the reasons were in your genes. You inherited longevity. Well, it's partly true that you inherit longevity. Living to 100 years old was once a genetic abnormality, a nice genetic abnormality but an abnormality nonetheless. People who lived to 100 stayed young much longer than other people. They worked longer and looked youthful. It turns out that genes kick in at the extremes of longevity and what has changed over time is where the 'extreme' starts. Getting to 100 once marked the extreme and was very unusual. It's much commoner now and in fact many babies born today can expect to have a lifespan into their 90s and beyond. The extreme has shifted to 105 or 110 – and research suggests those people do have healthy doses of longevity genes. What's pushed the extreme out to those ages, though, is how we live. Today, living well into your 90s has far less to do with your genes and more to do with what we can actually change in our lives, compared to what might have been only a generation or two ago.

Looking at the differences between identical and non-identical twins can tell a lot about the relative influence of genes compared to what we do to our bodies and the environment in which we live. If it's genetic, then identical twins will tend to show up in studies as being more similar to each other than fraternal twins.

A study of nearly 6000 twins in Denmark born in the late 19th century suggested that genes only contributed around 25 per cent towards longevity. The rest was environment, which includes lifestyle.

What really, really old people can teach us

#whilewearestillyoung
#genesarentdestiny (again)
#dontfester

Short of time? Living to over 100 is a stress test of your body, your lifestyle and the genes you were born with. It's a hurdle race which, the older you get, sifts out what matters in staying young longer because you've got rid of the 'noise' in the system. You'll find researchers confidently asserting they've found the genes that matter. But if you're looking for the one forever youthful gene, you'll be disappointed. The conundrum is that compared to the rest of us, really, really old people have similar patterns of genetic risk for Alzheimer's, heart disease and diabetes. It's just that they experience these problems later in life and probably have a few protective genes to help them along. In addition, the kind of person you are and how you respond to stress may count too. The bottom line, though, is that how and where you live count for a lot.

Okay … first things first: the statistics. At the moment, even in long-lived Japan, only around 4 people in every 10,000 are aged 100 or over, with Italy not far behind. By 2050, the proportion will have grown in both countries to around 4 people in every 1000. In Australia, the growth of centenarians (around 6 per cent each year) has been more than four times faster than general population growth and doesn't seem to be slowing down. Now, if living to 100 was a strongly genetic phenomenon, then you wouldn't expect such fast growth. You've got to look at people who are in their 60s to appreciate why the increase is happening and, to understand that, I need to digress to this thing called life expectancy.

Life expectancy is a misunderstood statistic.

It's usually referred to as the average number of years a newborn baby can expect to live. At the time of writing, an Australian baby can expect to live to age 83 give or take – longer for girls than boys. In 1900 life expectancy at birth was about 50.

The reasons for living longer have changed. You'd think, for instance, that if you were transported back 120 years, there would only be young and middle-aged people walking the streets of our cities. In fact, there would have been plenty of older people around because once you'd survived pregnancy, childhood and adolescence, you had a pretty good chance of getting to your 60s and 70s. The reason life expectancy was so low in the 19th century and beforehand was significantly due to the high mortality rate of children under the age of five, as well as the impact of women dying in pregnancy and childbirth. When a baby or young child dies, the numbers of years of life lost are huge. Years of life lost drag down life expectancy statistics and give a misleading idea of what the population looked like in those days.

In the 19th century, women became taller and better able to give birth safely. Childbirth itself became safer thanks to pioneers like Hungarian doctor Ignaz Semmelweis working in Vienna, who made medical students and doctors wash their hands before delivering babies and had his career and life destroyed by the virulent opposition his ideas generated. In the 1930s, by the way, even more gains in mothers surviving childbirth were made with the introduction of antibiotics. While obstetrics improved maternal and baby death rates, the really significant gains were due to the reduction of infectious (communicable) diseases in young kids. That meant gains in years of life which flowed through to life expectancy statistics. So what happened in the late 19th century and first half of the 20th century was that life expectancy went up because of a combination of factors: reductions in deaths from childhood infectious diseases due to immunisation, sanitation, food hygiene, better treatments for pneumonia and diarrhoea and the introduction of antibiotics, as well as the survival of mothers in pregnancy, labour and post-delivery. Societal factors also made the difference (see What the Taliban Know). In Australia in the 1920s, infectious diseases caused 15 per cent of deaths and the average age of those who died from an infection was 27 years. In Australia in 2018 – pre-COVID – infections caused 3 per cent of deaths and they largely affected people in their 80s and older.

So by 1950, life expectancy had increased to around the age of 65, mostly thanks to the increased number of years of life gained from improvements in the health of mothers, children and young adults. In fact, we'd pretty much maxed out life expectancy at birth in terms of the contribution from infection control and maternal and child health. If that's the case, though, how come we've added at least another 20 years life expectancy since then? Well, that's why you need to stop thinking about life expectancy at birth and shift to the idea of remaining life expectancy at various ages. You see, during the 50-odd years it took to raise life expectancy from 50 years to 65, the statistic that didn't change much from, say, around 1890 to just after World War 2, was your life expectancy at the age of 45 or 50, rather than at birth. In other words, if you were aged 45 in 1890 and aged 45 in 1950, you had a similar number of years left (about 20). What increased after 1950 in rich countries like Australia was our life expectancy at age 50 and, in fact, we've maxed out on that too and now the age at which remaining life expectancy is getting longer is 75.

Put another way, if you're 40 and reading this, then we pretty much know what's going to get you to your 90s unless you're run over by a truck or have genes that raise your risk of, say, heart disease or cancer and don't know you have them. We also know that these added years are generally healthy years worth having. You've got to work at it but you can get there in reasonably good shape.

The other thing that's important to know about the life expectancy statistic is that it's more than a simple average. It's actually a complex calculation based on what people die of today. It makes no allowances for the future. If you're aged 40, things will have changed a lot by the time you're 80 and, unless we're all hopelessly obese or in the middle of another pandemic or war, your chances of dying at age 80 are likely to be significantly reduced from what an 80-year-old faces today. Average life expectancy also doesn't account for being born into a well-off, well-educated family in an affluent suburb versus being born into disadvantage. A baby girl born today into well-off circumstances could have a lifespan well into her 90s, perhaps even into her 100s.

So what changed for 45-year-olds after World War 2? Well, income went up as did education and they make a difference. The more educated you are, the longer you live and the later in life you develop dementia, for instance. Prior to World War 2, being richer often meant you were fatter and looked 'prosperous' as they used to say. In the 1960s and later, being richer and better educated was associated with being thinner and healthier. Eventually the world realised how bad smoking was and people started to give up cigarettes. Our diets did get a bit healthier and GPs got better at recognising the risk factors for heart disease and stroke and had safe pills for lowering and controlling cholesterol and blood pressure. Modern medical technology had some impact with the ability of cardiologists and neurologists to save you from death and disability from heart attacks or strokes with clot-busting drugs and procedures to open up or replace blocked arteries. Some estimate the contribution of medical interventions versus prevention in cardiovascular disease reduction to be about 30 per cent. It turns out that stopping smoking has a large and immediate effect on your risk of premature death from heart attack and stroke, as does lowering your blood pressure and blood fats. Cancer death rates, adjusted for age, have also fallen, again more from prevention and early detection through screening than treatment which, apart from dramatic improvements in breast cancer and childhood leukaemia survival, has probably only shifted the dial on life expectancy by a little.

So all these things are making survival into our 90s and even to age 100 much more likely, thanks to prevention helped by medicine and surgery. Which means we have shifted the dial without changing our genes at all. What researchers argue, though, is that at whatever age we define as extreme old age (it was once reaching 100, now it's super-centenarians reaching 105 and beyond), genes do become more important. The trouble with the research into the genetics of ageing is that the studies are hard to do and often suffer from the small numbers of really, really old people (100+).

What we do know is that the super-old do share some common characteristics. For example, they're not obese or underweight, they're not smokers, have their blood pressure under control, and they usually have people they can call upon in times of trouble. But there's also a common psychological profile.

Personality plus: Tantalising evidence from large genetic studies suggests that there's a personality style which may be associated with a long life. Note I said 'associated' not necessarily cause and effect. It just may be that certain personality types are a sign of someone who may live longer than average – perhaps marking something else in them or their lives that's yet to be discovered. Even so, there are quite a few studies which suggest that people who are warm, conscientious, like being with people, look for stimulation in the world around them, and are more positive than others, tend to live longer lives. They're also less prone to anger, irritability, anxiety and depression. These personality traits are around 50 per cent inherited, which generally means our external environment makes up most of the other half. So these attributes are not totally fixed and it's possible to change and adapt your style of being in the world and if it doesn't lengthen your life, at least you'll be more pleasant to live with. Interestingly, a study of 5000 people in long-lived families, while confirming these personality traits in people who lived to extreme old age, found that they were also present in their husbands or wives, which suggests being nice is infectious or we choose people like us who may be nice people without necessarily needing genes to be so.

#getoverit: People who reach 100 and beyond also have an interesting way of dealing with stress. As Dr Margery Silver of the New England Centenarian Study told me a few years ago when I interviewed her at Harvard Medical School in Boston: 'They are able to manage stress very well. And this doesn't mean that they've had stress-free lives. Sometimes you think these people live so long, they must have had really easy lives; some of them have had really very difficult, and even traumatic lives. There are Holocaust survivors, there are women who were widowed at an early age and scrubbed floors to raise their children, and yet they seem to have the ability to roll with the punches.'

I asked Dr Silver to flesh out a bit more about how they respond to stress compared to other people.

'They don't ignore it,' she said. 'For instance, they're very good at handling losses, and they seem to accept their losses, grieve them and then move on. And in many situations solve a problem, recognise it's hard, and then move on. They bounce back.'

'They don't fester?'

'They don't fester.'

Based on that analysis of coping, I've got about five minutes left to live.

PART 1

Sweat the big stuff

#votelonglife

No time to lose: What determines how long the citizens of a nation live? Go on, tell me. What do you think? Sun and beaches? The national diet? How much they drive cars versus walking? The proximity to a fast-food outlet? Nope ... well, maybe yes to some of that, but you're getting into the weeds too quickly. Pull back the lens. A lot of it has to do with how we distribute the goodies.

Okay, quiz time.

Is it how much a nation spends on healthcare?

Not really. When you look at the league table of countries' life expectancies, it's true that longer-lived countries spend more on healthcare but that's an average. The famous example is the United States, which spends more than any other nation – by a long, long way – yet at the time of writing is number 46 on the league table with an average life expectancy of 79 years; while Japan, which is consistently either number one or two on life expectancy at 85 years, is down at 15th on how much it spends on healthcare.

So is it how rich a country is?

Well, it's certainly not good to be a low income nation but when you get above a certain level of per capita income, the link between how much a nation earns and how long its people live is loose. Qatar earns the most per head yet is 33rd on the life expectancy table. Australia is 21st on earnings yet is at number eight on life expectancy (again at the time of writing).

There are, however, some things which do stand out as being linked more strongly to how long the people of a nation live. One is the gap between rich and poor. Tragically, many poor nations have a wide divide between the wealthy and the poor but those where the gap is narrower do punch above their weight. Vietnam, for instance, is 126th on per capita income, yet has a narrower than average gap in income and rises to 84th in life expectancy. The United States has pretty wide income inequality and that's been getting worse, as has its global position on life expectancy.

This isn't about turning you into a Marxist Leninist revolutionary or a latter-day Robin Hood wanting to rob from the rich to give to the poor. It's about understanding what nations that have narrower income gaps tend to spend their money on and their attitudes to free markets which rely – crudely – on the rules of supply and demand and turning a profit. You see, free markets are great when you want to make and sell consumer products that people want to buy at the right price, but they don't work when it comes to goods like education and health which are essential for human development. Time and again it's been shown that, left to themselves, markets fail to provide education and health to those who have the least money. Markets can produce a cheaper car or piece of clothing but historically and in many different settings, they have been unable to provide for people who can't afford the prices of good education and healthcare, which are necessarily expensive to produce. Governments have to intervene to ensure quality, access and affordability, and that's what most upper-middle income and rich countries have done. Unless governments have their own independent sources of income, which is rare, it generally means taxing the rich disproportionately to the poor. It also means if politicians and bureaucrats care about how people live, they have to spend the money they receive in taxes on the areas where the market fails. So ... providing safe and effective healthcare (which usually means a focus on prevention and primary care) and high-quality education from early childhood, regardless of gender and ability to pay, are part of what's under the hood in nations that live long. Education level, for example, predicts how long you live, and whether and when you develop life-shortening conditions like heart disease, diabetes and dementia.

I know you want to jump ahead to see whether goji berries make you live longer but bear with me for a few minutes more.

This disconnect between a nation's economy and how long and well you live is only partial. A nation's average income per head of population does matter when it's desperately low. High quality healthcare and education are unaffordable when a country is poor, when poverty is rampant and basics such as food supply and clean air are not guaranteed. But the influence of average income per capita starts to disappear as the nation earns more and poverty and everything that goes with it is reduced. One measure is the human development index (HDI), which factors in three variables: a long and healthy life expectancy, which is a composite outcome of many factors such as breathing clean air, lifestyle opportunities, nutrition, smoking levels, the quality of work and access to healthcare. Secondly, how long people go on in education, and thirdly, gross national income (GNI) per capita. The HDI is simple – probably far too simple – and is biased towards countries that already have long life expectancies. In recent years, measures of poverty and gender inequality have been added, which help to explain differences in life expectancy independent of national income.

The point is, if you haven't already jumped to it, the most important politicians and bureaucracies determining how long the citizens of your nation live are Treasury and Finance, not Health (which in most governments should really be renamed Ministries of Illness). Treasury and Finance influence how national income is distributed and what investment is made in areas of market failure. If you had to choose the second-most important area of government, it would be Education and all too often that focuses on five-year-olds and older, missing out on what everyone but politicians and Finance bureaucrats know, which is that if you don't invest in a child's early years of education, you're struggling from the get-go.

There are many benefits of structured early childhood education in terms of employment and educational success but it does seem to have an effect on health in adulthood and by extension, longevity. Outside medicine, it's rare for social 'treatments' to undergo a randomised trial – meaning randomly allocating people to an intervention or a control. This has actually been done, though, in early childhood education. Two programs were offered to disadvantaged kids in North Carolina, from two months of age through to five years. These were subsequently adapted and implemented around the world, including Australia. Researchers followed up the original participants when they were in their mid-30s and what they found was extraordinary. When the participants were in their 30s there were significant benefits in income, BMI (obesity and overweight), cholesterol, smoking and blood pressure. If these were to be maintained until later in life, comparing those who went through the programs to those who didn't, there would be significant reductions in cancer, heart disease and stroke, and early deaths. A man aged 70 who went through one of these early childhood programs will likely have a quarter of the risk of dying at that age compared to a 70-year-old man who didn't. For those who went through the programs as young kids, it amounts to four years added to their lives without disabilities. For women, the effect is less but is still there. The message for cloistered economists in Treasury and Finance departments is that evidence-informed early childhood programs more than return taxpayers' investment.

Let me just take up a bit more of your time and pursue this a little longer because you can bang on about life-extending interventions at a microscopic level, when this big stuff has so much more impact in the population at large.

The Glasgow Effect – young lives matter

#younglivesmatter

Takeaway: Life expectancy is an average which hides stuff you need to know. The city I grew up in – Glasgow – to this day has a significant life expectancy gap between the best educated, wealthiest suburbs and the poorest – around 11 years. The country that's become my home – Australia – has an utterly shameful gap of 41 years between the longest and shortest-lived postcodes. Now, the easy assumption is that this is because fewer people who are aged 60 don't live to their 80s. That's partly true but the maths don't quite work because at age 60 there are too few years left to make a huge difference to the average life expectancy number (see my earlier explanation). The major reason for the life expectancy gap is that people die young instead of dying old and, as a result, a lot of years of life are lost. The causes, though, are different. When you die old, you're carted off by cancer, heart disease and dementia. When you die young, you die of self-harm, injury, violence, and alcohol and other drugs – the diseases of despair caused by poverty, thwarted opportunities and dislocation. Some have called this the Glasgow Effect.

Whenever I see a Safeway sign I get nauseous. It's nothing personal against Safeway which, I'm sure, is or was a perfectly fine chain of mass grocers. No, the reason is more ingrained. What the name evokes is a dreary, cold and wet Glaswegian Saturday afternoon when, aged around ten years old, I've been dragged to do the weekly supermarket shopping with my mum in the family's rusting Ford Anglia. The ineffectual heater is on, the windows are closed and misting up, and my mother is smoking one fag after the other. Today that'd be cause for accusations of child neglect but back then it was standard operational procedure for parents.

The West of Scotland – which mostly means Glasgow – has higher rates of dying young (premature mortality) than other parts of Scotland and indeed many other parts of Britain and Europe. A man living in Dennistoun, a suburb with high levels of deprivation, has only a 53 per cent chance of living to the age of 65. The easily assumed explanation is drinking, smoking, lack of exercise and fried Mars bars, but it goes deeper than that and has lessons for us all in terms of living young longer.

Sir Harry Burns is Professor of Global Public Health at Strathclyde University in Glasgow. He's a former surgeon who converted to public health and for several years was Scotland's Chief Medical Officer. He told me: 'If you look at the trends in life expectancy, it's only really in the past few decades that our improvement in life expectancy has slowed down. And when you look even further it's slowed down largely because the growth in life expectancy in the poorest sectors of the population has slowed down a lot.'

Paradoxically, if you're better off and living in Glasgow, your life expectancy is going up faster than the European average. 'The gap in life expectancy between rich and poor has always existed, but it began to widen very substantially probably in the 1960s,' claimed Professor Burns. 'And if you look at what was happening at that time, you could see disintegration of communities as post-war housing booms started to take over.

The old tenement buildings in Glasgow were being knocked down, and they should have been knocked down because they were no longer fit for human habitation, there were outside toilets and so on. But what replaced them did not facilitate community connectedness. People supported each other because they were all living in the same circumstances. But suddenly people were being spread all over the West of Scotland because there was a fashion for building new towns.'

Sure, smoking rates and a lousy diet were and are a problem but again, paradoxically, not much more of a problem in Glasgow than other areas of deprivation in Britain. The impact has been greatest in the young. According to Harry Burns: 'If you die of a drugs overdose, typically you'll do that when you're young, so you might miss out on 50 or 60 years worth of life expectancy. And when you calculate life expectancy, a death at 25 is significantly more impactful than a death at 75. Poor people in their 20s and 30s and 40s are far more likely to die than more affluent people of the same age. And that seems to be what's driving the gap in life expectancy, not deaths at a later age.'

So what's the full explanation, because when you look at the immediate causes they're injury, drug and alcohol. People born in the 1960s during the maximal time of dislocation seem to be most at risk of early death. Their parents had lost their jobs and, in many ways, their identities and social supports and this flowed on to their kids. It's almost like a deadly social and economic contagion which is then passed on to the next generation both socially and genetically. (See Get Out of Those Genes.)

'There is some evidence that there is some genetic switching going on in children who experience stressful childhoods,' said Professor Burns, who assisted colleagues to set up a program focused on very young children. It's called the Early Years Collaborative, involving hundreds of people working in childhood services as well as many local authorities across Scotland who come together regularly to learn from one another's experiences. The Collaborative's projects include simple programs such as encouraging parents to read more bedtime stories to their kids.

There are lessons for us all from this because step one in living young is being allowed to live young.

What the Taliban know

#whatdotheyknow? That when you educate women, the world changes.

#whatdonttheyknow? That when you educate women, Taliban men will live longer, healthier lives. Trouble for Taliban men is that women will live longer too.

Keep paddling up the stream for the answers (because downstream you get stuck in the weeds): Quite a few years ago, while I was making a Channel 4 (UK) television series on the origins of disease, I was warned by a researcher I trusted to keep my eyes and ears open because, for example, if I thought that the real causes of heart disease were cholesterol and smoking, it was going to be a very disappointing series. What he was referring to was what in public health they call the 'upstream' causes of living short and living long. He told me to go and see Barry Smith – the late Professor Francis Barrymore Smith, a Melbourne and Cambridge trained historian – which I did, and was told an amazing story.

One of the terrible life-shortening diseases of the 19th and 20th centuries was (and still is in low income countries) tuberculosis (TB), a bacterial infection which can affect almost any organ in the body, particularly the lungs. I've no idea whether you're an opera-goer but it was what sent off Mimi in *La Bohème* and knocked down Nicole Kidman (Mimi's meme) in Baz Luhrmann's *Moulin Rouge*, both set in Paris in the 19th century.

I'll get to the Taliban in a minute. I'm telling you this story to begin with to illustrate how, if you want to live young long, don't make assumptions too quickly.

They'll deny it, but the physicians and surgeons who treat disease have long been in a battle with the doctors and researchers who want to prevent us having shorter, less happy lives. If you doubt this, just look at the money that goes into hospitals, drugs and things that go *'ping'* versus the invisible stuff that keeps us young.

Anyway, tuberculosis was once their battlefield and its history was Barry Smith's special interest.

The prevention people (public health) liked to say that the treatment side of medicine only contributed maybe 10 per cent to the gains in life expectancy seen in the 19th and first half of the 20th century. It was what the public health people did in terms of clean water and air and less hunger that made the difference. The curative doctors fought back over TB. They'd noticed TB was declining and claimed the triumph was medical science, which had developed anti-TB medications such as one called streptomycin. The public health people countered and said while it was true that TB was declining, its rates were falling long before streptomycin and it was what they did with sanitation and better housing and nutrition in the 19th century that made the difference.

Barry Smith argued that most of the decline had occurred before a lot of these measures had kicked in. It's a difficult story to disentangle because there was a lot happening at the same time. There were improvements in housing, nutrition and reductions in deprivation, as well as measures well known to us in the times of COVID, namely detecting cases and isolating them (when possible) to stop spread. But Smith and colleagues found parishes in Europe which appeared to have less TB than parishes which looked pretty similar in terms of poverty and levels of deprivation.

Their finding was that the parishes with less TB were the ones which taught girls to read and write.

Have you ever wondered why the Taliban and their fellow mediaeval fundamentalists are so opposed to young girls going to school that they'll take murderous action against teachers and students? The answer can be found in the research of Australian demographer Professor Jack Caldwell, who wondered what were the key determinants of poor countries which became successful in terms of living healthier and longer lives.

The technical way of expressing this is the transition that nations make from high mortality to low mortality – moving from dying young to dying old.

Jack Caldwell, who died in 2016, was, in his day, arguably the leading researcher in his field worldwide. He and his wife Pat, who was often his co-researcher, were fascinated by the process of poor countries transitioning to middle income and low mortality and what happened to women in that process. Caldwell was critical of the role of religion in holding back development in low income countries, although he acknowledged that wasn't always the case. He (and others) found that regardless of the availability of contraception, as family wealth increased, the numbers of children they had decreased. The reasons were complex and had to do with no longer having to rely on children as family labourers for income as much as in the past.

But it was also related to women's autonomy and where *that* came from, according to Jack and Pat Caldwell, was education.

Teaching little girls to read and write was and is transformative.

At a time when the assumption was that all that needed to happen for people to live longer healthier lives was for nations to make more money, Caldwell noticed a paradox. Kerala in India, Sri Lanka and Costa Rica all seemed to have made a transition from dying young to dying older, at a time when their per capita income hadn't changed much. In other words, they were just as poor as many other nations yet for some reason they were living longer. In fact, they had similar life expectancies to much richer nations.

There were a few things going on to explain this.

Women had higher levels of education than similarly poor nations. They had more power in their communities and there was more investment in health at the level of families, to look after mothers and their kids. Well, you might say, the key is that women were in charge and that it wasn't necessarily education. However, there's been plenty of other research in less matriarchal cultures to show that women's education in its own right is powerfully linked to living longer and, in fact, is a much stronger influence than national income once a country lifts itself out of desperate poverty. It's been estimated that a 10 per cent gain in the level of literacy has four times the effect on extra years of life expectancy than a 10 per cent gain in national income.

And, by the way, Taliban take note: when women are educated, males benefit more than women from this gain in years of healthy life.

So what is it about women's education that makes the difference? Well, this is what the Taliban *do* know.

Caldwell and others concluded that a lot of it has to do with the increased autonomy that women get when they can read and write, learn maths and proceed to higher education if it's available. Family income goes up and demand for basic healthcare does too.

Very threatening if you have narrow, fundamentalist views of religions and their teachings.

Mind you

#itsallone

Quick one: This is a section largely for millennials and younger because mental health issues usually start when you're young. But anyway, you know the story already: healthy body, healthy mind etc. However, you can't repeat often enough that there's no separation between what goes on inside your skull – your brain/mind – and the rest of your body. So it shouldn't be a shock revelation that if things are going well with your mood and your level of psychological strain and stress, as reflected in how much control you feel you have over your life, it'll have an impact on your arteries, heart, gut and your capacity to keep yourself young.

Psychological wellbeing buys you years. Conversely, mental ill health can cost you years and I say that not to panic you but to encourage anyone with mental health issues to seek help.

Some of the best data on this come from Denmark, where they have superb records and disease registers which allow realistic measures of the life expectancy impact of psychological issues. Researchers followed more than 7 million people for a total of more than 111 million person years. The good news is that their findings show that the impact of mental health is less than previously thought but it's still significant. The chances of dying younger than you would otherwise were two-fold higher for people with depression and anxiety and up to a four-fold increase for people with a drug or alcohol problem. When you measure this in terms of years of life lost, dying young obviously has a bigger impact. It's what I've said a couple of times already: namely, a death when someone's in their 30s loses more years of life. I tell you this because intervening when you're young is very important. Don't wait to get this stuff sorted out.

I'm about to translate that into years of life lost but remember these are averages. It's not your unalterable destiny so therefore it's changeable.

The Danish analysis found that the worst life-shortening problem was substance use to the extent that it had become a disorder. That shortened a person's remaining time by an astounding 13–15 years. The effect of depression and anxiety was a loss of 6–8 years, while people diagnosed with schizophrenia potentially lost 9–12 years. Now, you probably think these years of life are lost because of suicide but in fact the main reasons are the physical illnesses which affect people with mental health issues. It's more about cancer, heart disease and diabetes.

The reasons depend on the severity of the psychological issue a person has but include unemployment, lack of somewhere to live, high smoking rates, low levels of physical activity, poor nutrition, medication side effects, psychiatrists who forget they're doctors and behave as though the mind and body are separate and don't attend to the physical health of their patients, and stigma from the healthcare system which can neglect to give people with mental illness the general medical care they need.

The commonest issues relate to psychological distress, which is partly related to depression and anxiety. The ways psychological distress manifests itself include having little interest or pleasure in doing things; feeling down, depressed or hopeless; having trouble falling or staying asleep or sleeping too much; feeling tired or having too little energy; your appetite is poor or you're overeating; you're feeling bad about yourself, or that you're a failure and have let yourself or your family down; you have trouble concentrating on things; people are noticing you're moving around more slowly than usual or the opposite, being so fidgety or restless that you're moving around a lot more; and having thoughts that you would be better off dead – or hurting yourself in some way – which is a flashing red light that you need help straight away.

However, in some people, distress and depression and anxiety show up more as persistent physical symptoms like fatigue, disruption of your sleep–wake cycle, pain, headaches and tummy symptoms.

One way of deciding whether you need to seek help is whether your work is being affected, you've lost the ability to complete tasks, damaged your personal and family relationships, and/or are no longer pursuing your interests and involvement with friends.

When you're distressed, using tobacco, alcohol and other drugs to try to make you feel better is a really bad idea. The effects are short lived and the harms – like having a shorter life – are more profound.

The treatment for distress is usually a stepped approach depending on the severity, urgency and your preference. It starts with simple lifestyle changes – such as sleep, diet, exercise and reduction of alcohol – then basic problem solving, stress management and life skills, and if these aren't working, moving on to more specialised psychological therapies and, if necessary, medication.

Get out of those genes

#knowyourfamily

Quick take: I know it sounds morbid, but it's handy to know what your family dies of and when. Yes, I know I said earlier

32

that genes only take you so far in living young into old age, but there are some genes that get in the way and can mean you risk dying young unless you do something about it. This, by the way, isn't a sell-job to go off and have your genes sequenced because while a lot is known about genetic risk, there are still huge swathes of unknowns. Bottom line is that it's useful to be aware of who died of what and when in your family. If there is a pattern of people dying young or being diagnosed with, say, heart disease or cancer under the age of 50 (some would say 60), particularly in first and second degree relatives, then you too are potentially at risk and need to have a close look with your GP and perhaps genetic specialists to find ways of getting out of those genes with lifestyle changes or medical screening aimed at early diagnosis and treatment. Rather than a cheap set of mail-order gene tests, if there is a pattern in your family of premature death, what's more useful is asking your doctor to refer you for genetic counselling. Often, targeted gene testing can show that you don't have to worry and sometimes you may think there's a familial problem when there isn't.

When I was a medical student I was an A-grade hypochondriac. In my defence it was because there seemed to be a lot of cancer in my family: an uncle, three grandparents and other relatives. My most shameful episode was one afternoon in third year studying in the pathology museum for my exam the next day. Most medical schools in those days had pathology museums, which were filled with large glass or perspex jars containing specimens of some organ or other taken from a hapless patient during an operation or, even more morbidly, at an autopsy.

During the pathology exam, you'd be given one of these 'pots', as they were known, and had to diagnose it and talk about the condition. So I was cramming pots. Anyway, the sample in front of me was of an osteosarcoma, a rare-ish bone cancer. The pot contained a tibia – the large bone of the lower leg – and it harboured an osteosarcoma from someone who'd had the disease below the knee.

As I read the textbook description of osteosarcoma and how it presented and the poor survival rates – they're much better these days – my hand drifted to my own tibia, the left one. I froze in horror. My blood instantly chilled to sub-zero. My mouth suddenly became dry as a bone (so to speak). What I'd come across was a painless, bony lump just below my knee. I frantically looked at the textbook again. I was in the peak age group. I looked at the pot. This could be my tibia in a future pot being examined by a future medical student who'd have no idea it had belonged to a genius cut down before his prime.

In a trance I got up and walked across to the hospital and straight to the office of the professor of orthopaedic surgery, planning what I'd do with my last days and how I'd tell my mum and dad. The professor was in his office and for some reason his secretary let me in. Must have been the panic on my face. He looked up and brusquely (well, he was an orthopaedic surgeon) asked why I was there. I blurted out the story and I think I actually said that why I was there was to find out how long I had left.

A knowing expression came across his face and he asked me to lie on the examination bed and show him the lump. He studiously felt it – and keeping a completely straight face – said, 'Yes, you do have a lump there, but would you like to feel your right tibia? There's one just like it there.' I should have been thrown out of medical school there and then. What I'd felt was normal. My lump was an anatomical protrusion called the tibial tuberosity. But I was too stupid to feel embarrassed or shamed by this.

I actually walked out of his office on air (no doubt he was shaking his head behind my back). I was floating. I had my life back. It took maybe an hour or two to start worrying if the professor of orthopaedics had rung the professor of pathology warning him of this nutter they'd be seeing in the next day's exam.

I'm not going to write a textbook of genetics for you (what I truly know about genetics can be written on the back of one of the smaller chromosomes) but will give you a general idea. While I know you can't wait for me to get on to red wine, anti-ageing drugs and, yes, goji berries, carrying potentially life-shortening genes is something you'd best know about because there are usually things you can do to work around the genetic hand those parents and grandparents of yours have dealt you.

First thing to say is that while it's important to know if there are patterns of disease in your family which suggest there are problematic genes, some people are the first in their family to develop a genetic disorder, either because of a new mutation or because the rogue gene has been silent for a generation or more and, for some reason, reveals itself and manifests in a single family member.

Let's start with patterns which suggest you might have an inherited risk of cancer. I'll get to heart disease in a minute.

One pattern is that three or more members of your family have had one of a range of cancers which include (most commonly) bowel, uterus, ovary, stomach, liver/gallbladder, kidney, brain and some skin cancers; also in this pattern is that two or more successive generations of your family have been affected; and lastly, that at least one of your family has been diagnosed with one of these tumours before the age of 50. This pattern is called 'Lynch syndrome' and is probably the commonest inherited cancer syndrome. Lynch syndrome is caused by a failure of the cells in your body to correct errors in your DNA and there are genetic tests which can be done after you've had genetic counselling. One of the reasons for the counselling is to understand your risk status, the process of testing, what to expect and, if negative, reassure you. You also may not have Lynch but could have another genetic syndrome which needs to be investigated. If you test positive then you can set up a surveillance/early detection process with your doctors since, for most cancers, the best chance of cure is to find the tumour early.

Another pattern which is commonest in women but can occur in men also involves a range of cancers but primarily breast and ovarian cancer. Sorry, this is going to be complicated but it's important to know.

The pattern includes a family history of:

* Breast cancer diagnosed under the age of 50
* Breast cancer in someone who has Ashkenazi Jewish ancestry
* Two or more relatives with breast cancer if one has been diagnosed younger than 50
* Three or more relatives with breast cancer at any age, ovarian cancer usually at a younger age

* A particular kind of breast cancer called triple negative – not having receptors (lock and key mechanisms) to the two female hormones oestrogen and progesterone and a cell growth factor called HER2 – under the age of 60
* Pancreas and prostate cancer in families who also have a history of breast cancer
* Multiple primary related cancers happening in the same family member

This pattern is typical of mutations in genes called BRCA1 and BRCA2 and needs a referral for genetic counselling and testing.

Some people have strong family histories of cancer yet have no recognisable mutation or gene pattern when genetically tested. That doesn't mean you don't have a familial risk, and you should take care to be checked at regular intervals for early detection. With ovarian cancer, at the time of writing, there really isn't a reliable screening test and the diagnosis usually requires removal of the ovary and fallopian tubes. So what some women opt for is prophylactic removal of their breasts and ovaries in a careful decision-making process with their specialist.

If a woman with no family history of cancer is having her tubes tied, it's worth asking the gynaecologist what she thinks about removing the part of the fallopian tubes nearest the ovary as this is where some ovarian cancers may begin. This simple procedure may be lifesaving and preserve the ovaries. This is NOT a solution for women with a genetic risk of ovarian cancer.

Prostate cancer can be hereditary too in its own right and a signal is a first-degree relative with prostate cancer (brother, son or father), particularly but not necessarily if diagnosed at a young age. And like the other familial cancers, you might need genetic counselling to check there isn't a risk of other cancers in, say, the female members of your family and find out what surveillance you might need. In fact, a family history of prostate cancer or indeed pancreatic cancer in men can be a sign that the person who's transmitted the BRCA gene is the father. Men carrying BRCA mutations need surveillance too, including for male breast cancer and a heightened awareness of the risks of stomach and prostate cancer. Surveillance for pancreatic cancer is controversial but important since it is a nasty tumour. Researchers are encouraging doctors to look for warning signs. Professor Rachel Neale of the Queensland Institute of Medical Research told me, 'There are things like somebody who is aged over 50 or 40 who has a new diagnosis of diabetes ... We do know that new onset diabetes can be a red flag in some people, so that would be an example where you put things together.'

Another symptom is pain in the upper abdomen that's typical of what's called biliary pain. Rachel Neale again: 'Experienced GPs are able to distinguish between epigastric pain and biliary type pain, and particularly biliary type pain gets worse after ingestion of fat or a heavy meal, and that's more likely to be something like gallstones than it is pancreatic cancer. So it's important that GPs are able to distinguish between different types of pain and explore those.'

Then the question is: what test to have done? Some gastroenterologists have expertise in a procedure called 'endoscopic ultrasound', where they do an endoscopy and from inside the upper intestinal tract do an ultrasound of the pancreas, looking for lumps and nodules. Most experts, though, think a CT scan focusing on the pancreas (pancreatic protocol) is a better, less invasive procedure. The trouble is that it's not clear what to do if they find a benign nodule since it may never turn into a cancer and surgery of the pancreas is complex and needs a highly skilled hepatobiliary surgeon to carry it out.

Heart disease is hugely an environmental condition caused by diet, inactivity, smoking and diabesity (diabetes and obesity) but it can run in families. Having had a childhood and adolescence in Glasgow, with a chip-pan on the cooker for our twice daily hit of hot fat and calories and many afternoons spent in smoke-filled sitting-rooms with my great-aunties, I'm sure the environment has overwhelmed my genes. But here are some patterns that might indicate a familial risk of heart disease.

One is having a brother, sister, parent or son/daughter diagnosed with heart disease under the age of 55 in men and under the age of 65 in women. Another is a family history of heart disease in association with a family history of stroke and/or diabetes. A third is a family history of sudden cardiac death particularly at an early age as, in addition to coronary heart disease, this can indicate a familial risk of what are called 'cardiomyopathies', which are diseases of the heart muscle. Abnormal heart rhythms can also be familial, sometimes caused by a cardiomyopathy. Some people are born with heart defects (congenital heart disease) and sometimes they can be familial. While congenital heart disease used to be almost exclusively a childhood problem, with better care kids with congenital heart disease are surviving into adulthood and often need specialised care.

Noticing a familial pattern of heart disease can save your life or someone's in your family and help you or them to die old instead of young. Simple tests include your cholesterol (familial high cholesterol levels are commoner than you might think and very treatable), echocardiography (heart ultrasound) and chest X-rays, and there's also other more sophisticated testing.

The main message in all this is that it's better to know.

Me ... this long-term survivor of hypochondriasis – as I write this I'm on bowel prep for my colonoscopy tomorrow, so you should be glad I was able to squeeze out this section.

Is what you see what you get?

#lookingood
#rollingstonegathersnomoss

First impressions: If you look young on the outside, are you young on the inside? And could it be that looking good indicates you'll live longer? According to some research, yes. If you look younger, you may well have made a greater effort to keep fit and healthy, giving you a greater chance of living younger longer. But there may be deeper biology going on. For example, sun damage is more than skin deep. It affects the rest of your body. Plastic surgery messes with this a little but we'll come to that. Bottom line is that how old you are on the inside and outside is what counts and the aim is to keep your age lower than how old your birth certificate says you are.

Oh, would some Power give us the gift
To see ourselves as others see us!
It would from many a blunder free us,
And foolish notion:
What airs in dress and gait would leave us,
And even devotion!
'To A Louse' – Robert Burns

Burns, the 18th century Scottish bard, knew all about appearances and the falsity of airs and graces, seeing right through them. In this poem he was writing about a wee beastie that was crawling – unnoticed – on an uppity lady's bonnet in church. The louse doesn't understand that its host is an important person, and could be shamed by the indignity of a fellow villager watching it wandering about. His point was that humans will never have the luxury of the louse. We cannot see ourselves as others see us. It's central to the human condition.

We think we know the way we look, the way we present to others. Social media has made some of us even more obsessed about image and appearance because there's always that unknown, that element of uncertainty about how we're perceived by friends, family and strangers. Burns knew that appearances and context are bound together. In modern terms, it comes down to class, religion, gender and … biology. The way you look may reflect how long you're going to live in good health but it's not a one-way street. You can back up a bit.

Skin deep? The exception proves the rule, they say, and there can be no more public exception when it comes to appearances and ageing than Rolling Stones guitarist Keith Richards. At the time of writing, he's still kicking away at close to 80, despite having looked as though he's been 80 years old for decades.

Most of us aren't Keith Richards and don't have what he has, which is clearly the constitution of an ox. Looking young reflects good body maintenance and therefore a greater chance of biological youth, and there is research to support the notion that your appearance can predict how long you live.

One study was from a long-term follow-up of same-sex twins in Denmark, slightly over half of whom were identical. The twins were aged between 70 and 99 when they'd had high quality digital colour head shot photos taken, as well as a host of other measures. What the researchers wanted to know was whether people's perceptions of the age of a person from how they looked correlated with their chronological age and physical measures of biological age, such as thinking and memory (cognitive function), muscular strength as measured by the power of their grip, performance on stair climbing and the length of their telomeres – those ageing clocks at the end of our chromosomes. Three kinds of assessor were used to see how generalisable were the perceptions: experienced geriatric nurses; young, male student teachers (who were expected to be lousy at the task); and women in their 70s and 80s (that is, roughly the same age as the twins being studied).

Regardless of whether the assessor was an expert (the geriatric nurses) or one of the others, their rating of perceived age closely correlated with other measures of the twins' biological age. In other words, if they looked old, they were weaker, had shorter telomeres and had more issues with cognitive function. The older 'peer' women, interestingly, over-rated the twins' ages by nearly two years.

In a seven-year follow-up, the chances of a twin dying sooner than their sibling were significantly higher in those who were perceived to be older (and probably, in fact, were biologically older).

Put another way, those deemed to look younger lived longer.

There seems to be a genetic contribution to this, since identical twins showed the effect more strongly than non-identical twins. However, the environment clearly plays a role since there is other research which shows that your perceived age from how you look is related to whether you smoke, have been overexposed to the sun, have had depression, and your socioeconomic status (the tougher your life, the older your perceived age).

When you look at some of the factors that make you appear older, it starts to make sense.

Smoking: Tobacco smoke is one of the strongest pro-oxidants known. It causes oxidative stress and inflammation throughout the body, ageing your brain, your arteries, your heart, your kidneys and your skin.

Sun: Ultraviolet light from the sun causes damage and oxidative stress in the dermis – the substructure of the skin – causing deep wrinkling, abnormal pigmentation, widening of tiny blood vessels making them visible (telangiectasia) and a 'sallow' complexion. The damage also triggers the innate immune system (see Anna Karenina and the Microbiome), which means that white blood cells travel to the skin to see what's going on, become activated then travel to other parts of the body, passing on the inflammation they've learned from sun-damaged skin.

Socioeconomic status: That relates to where you live, your exposure to air pollution, your ability to afford a decent diet, and chronic stress.

Depression: There is a reasonable body of evidence that depression brings on an inflammatory and therefore pro-ageing state.

Cellular senescence: One of the causes and signs of ageing is that some cells stop working and instead of being eliminated, they hang around causing trouble. There is evidence that old looking skin contains senescent cells which may reflect their existence elsewhere in the body (see Putting Out the Garbage).

Bottom line: You don't want anyone saying you look older than you are because this study showed that you don't need to be a medical expert to tell that. On the other hand, you should be tickled pink if someone says you look young for your age.

Biological age vs what's on the clock

#cuttingthebull

Just about the best fun I've ever had on television was during the several seasons I did as medical host on *The Biggest Loser.* I learned there was nothing real about reality television. Duuh, you might say. Anyway, if you never watched it, the idea is that 15 to 20 very obese people get locked away in a seemingly isolated location for several months with a group of experienced trainers – like Michelle Bridges and 'Commando' Steve Willis. The contestants lived together and went through a gruelling program of calorie restriction, nutritional education and calorie burning through aerobic and strength training. Like most reality shows, contestants get progressively eliminated until you end up with the newly and miraculously lithe biggest loser – literally. A couple of former ABC TV colleagues who worked on *The Biggest Loser* approached me to do it. They actually wanted me to become the Biggest Bastard on *The Biggest Loser*, which I refused to do, and we eventually came to a deal where I'd go along with some of the showbiz requirements of commercial television in return for which I'd get to communicate some quite complex concepts about health and wellbeing to an audience that I didn't normally have access to through the ABC. While the show had lots of critics as being unrealistic and unsustainable, it did do some good. We conducted a whole-town series in Ararat in regional Victoria, one of the fattest places in Australia. The population of Ararat lost an average of more than 3 kg each during the weeks of the show, which is an enormous public health result.

Anyway, back on set, there were many paradoxes and ironies behind the scenes. One was that the production company that made *The Biggest Loser* was the same one that made *MasterChef* and they used the same crew caterers, whose food had to be good enough to appeal to the celebrity chefs on *MasterChef*. So at lunch we'd very guiltily eat five-star food while the unknowing contestants went back for a carrot.

The first show I did, the producers wanted to do DEXA scans on the participants. In medicine, DEXA scans are used to assess bone density in the diagnosis of osteoporosis. In elite sport, though, DEXA scans measure body composition because the scan can differentiate fat from muscle from bone. I was really unhappy because I didn't want viewers to rush out and ask their GP for a DEXA scan. The producers – as they do in television – thought the pictures would be great. We came to a compromise. I agreed with the use of DEXA scans as long as they'd let me do the evidence-based measure, which is waist circumference. The producers were right. The scans were amazing because they could build up the picture of the person's body from the skeleton outwards. When you're carrying a lot of weight, your skeleton looks pretty robust – it needs to be. There's a lot to support. Then they superimposed the muscles and many obese people have reasonable musculature for the same reason. So at the stage where you're showing the skeleton and muscles, the person actually looks a bit like Commando. Then comes the fat and the person turns into a sphere. *The Biggest Loser* contestants that year were 53 per cent fat.

Next was measuring waist circumference.

Now, I trained in paediatrics. I've never been a general practitioner and when GPs hear this story they either take pity or laugh at my ignorance. We got one of the contestants up on the stage. There were six cameras and we were filming 'as live' so there was a degree of stress. I had thought it was going to be easy. One of the producers who was much smarter than me had acquired a 'bariatric' tape measure, which was longer than average. Meanwhile I hadn't worked out how to do this, although the producers assumed I had. I thought I'd put my arms around the contestant's waist and catch the tape behind his back. This is the point that experienced GPs start to groan. Not on your nelly. I ended up getting the poor guy to hold one end of the tape while I walked round him with the other. In so doing, I made a discovery. Obesity doesn't make you spherical. It makes you oval. In old units he was 5 feet 8 inches tall and 6 feet around the waist. For all its flaws, when the contestants came on to the show they had diabetes, high blood pressure and many other issues, which had largely disappeared by the end.

Why am I telling you all this? Well, one of the most popular segments was when we used a proprietary program to assess contestants' biological age compared to how old they were chronologically. After a couple of series, new contestants knew what to expect and they started to cry as soon as I walked out onto the set, before I'd said a word. Good for reality television 'moments' but crap for the ego. Numbers flashing up on a big screen kind of indicated their progress to premature death if they didn't do anything, and the bio-age segment ended up being quite a motivator. I'm not going to use their measures of biological age because this whole area is controversial, but there are factors which predict that you will lose years of life and years of healthy life.

There are many markers of being biologically older than your calendar age. High blood pressure, high blood sugars and fats, too big a waist circumference (it needs to be a LOT less than 2 metres), resting pulse rate, exercise tolerance, muscle strength, cognitive impairment, and levels of chronic stress and psychological distress are all markers of increased biological age and I'll get to them later. There are also cellular markers such as having shorter telomeres – the protective bits at the ends of your chromosomes and something called DNA methylation – a chemical reaction in your DNA which can change how well your genes work despite there being no mutation. It's known as the epigenetic clock.

I've already mentioned the significance of how old you look compared to your chronological age. Looking older than you should could indicate internal organ ageing. If you recognise this young enough, you could do a lifestyle audit using the information in this book to intervene. The aim is to reduce oxidative stress – biological rusting – and restore your metabolic balance – homeostasis – so that it's less tilted towards ageing.

I want to say more about this balance/homeostasis thing, which is a recurring theme in this book, because it's an important factor in ageing and helps to explain why it's hard but far from impossible to slow ageing down and sometimes even to reverse it.

The balance thing – why what's good for you can be bad for you

#watchyourkilter

Quick take: What's good for you can be bad for you and what seems to be bad for you can sometimes be good for you. Our bodies work best when there's a balance and the challenge of staying young as long as possible is restoring the balance to a youthful profile. It's bloody frustrating but there is a way through.

Apologies ahead of time if you see this message repeated in various parts of the book, but it needs to be, because this issue of balance – called homeostasis – is really at the heart of why our bodies change as the years go by.

Just about every process that keeps us alive has a counterforce. We store fat and we can bring it out of stores. The same goes for sugar (glucose). The system that raises our blood pressure can lower it. When free radicals are produced and start to damage and age our muscles, heart, brain, immune system and kidneys, the same system can dampen down this oxidative stress. And so on. Think about this balance as being a bit like a rocket ship going straight up when we're biologically young. When we start to age, the balance loses some control and the trajectory is tilted to one side so the rocket starts to fly in a different direction. Trouble is that all the on-board mechanisms and steering readjust themselves to the new direction and stubbornly resist attempts to fly straight up. The tilt – the abnormal homeostasis – becomes the new normal.

It happens in cancer too. The body's homeostatic control of cell growth gets tilted towards growth, and so powerful is the new homeostasis that attempts to shift it back with chemo and radiation often fail. That's one reason why cancer treatments often involve using drug combinations, namely to unbalance the new balance.

I want you to keep this in mind as you read on because some anti-ageing interventions don't seem to work when all the research in the lab suggests they should. The problem is that the way these compounds are used at the moment is not enough to shift this huge rocket back on track. And they may not be given in the right dose. The interventions we know do work attack ageing on multiple fronts, sometimes at surprisingly low doses.

More is not necessarily better: We tend to think about drugs, for example, having the same basic effect on the body regardless of dose. So raising the dose just makes it more effective as long as you don't get side effects but that's not necessarily true. The mind-twisting notion behind saying that more isn't necessarily better is that some substances have entirely different effects at low doses than at high doses. Take smoking, for instance. The first ten cigarettes a day are much more toxic than the next ten.

It's not a straight line. Normal doses of oxygen are good for us in the air we breathe but high doses can be toxic.

On the other hand, low doses of bioactive substances in our diet may activate protective pathways whereas high doses may overwhelm them and throw out the balance in a bad direction. Vitamins are the classic example; we seem happy to take massive amounts of vitamin supplements in the belief that more is better when, in fact, high doses may work against us. For instance, there's evidence that high dose vitamin C supplements can be pro-ageing.

Some researchers call this paradox 'adaptive homeostasis'. Our bodies are battle hardened from millennia of evolution to adapt to adversity and, once they do, it's hard to shift these adaptations. That's one of the secrets of survival. Ageing is a form of adaptive homeostasis – some would say maladaptive – but we've got to be careful how we shift it back because we could do it too bluntly and suffer untoward consequences. Ageing research suffers from a focus on single substances which are probably not enough to tip us back to a youthful balance, or maybe they're being given in the wrong dose, or maybe they're inadvertently setting us up for other problems.

So be careful what you wish for. (You'll hear that one again too.)

Where's reverse on the human gearshift?

#showustheclutch

Quick park: This is a core debate among researchers into ageing. Not so much about whether you can reverse ageing, because the evidence suggests that, for example, you can rejuvenate your muscles with reasonably intense muscle strengthening – at any age. You can stimulate nerve growth and new connections in the brain – again with fairly intensive exercise and maybe even dietary restriction. You could also argue that even some medical procedures like coronary stents to open up blocked arteries are artificially returning a bit of youth to the heart. If you add that to the bioactives you consume in a highly diverse, plant-dominated cuisine, and the promise of all kinds of anti-ageing medications and supplements (see Which Pill and Why?), it's pretty clear you can live younger. The question is whether that necessarily means you live longer. The sum of the evidence pretty powerfully suggests that yes, you can, but there are still scientists who think we're reaching our limit.

To follow this argument and come to your own conclusion, there are a few things to clarify. The first is not to confuse what happens at a population level with what each of us as individuals can achieve. I've alluded to this already. Saying that the life expectancy of Australians is around 83 years of age hides a lot of detail that matters. Now what I'm about to say repeats what I said earlier, but it's worth emphasising because it's easy to assume that 'life expectancy' is a forecast of what to expect in the future. It isn't. It's a snapshot average based on *this year's* calculations of births and deaths and what are called 'life tables'. Here are some of the things that it hides. One is that a baby born today in an advantaged suburb could well live to 100. Even in disadvantaged postcodes, if a baby gets through the early years and middle age, they too can live to a ripe old age. I talked about this in the Glasgow Effect. When we refer to gaps in average life expectancy between rich and poor, these differences aren't so much because people are dying at 70 instead of 85. It's that young people are dying. When someone dies in their 30s or 40s of suicide, injury or drug and alcohol complications, putting aside the tragedy, the impact of all these years of life lost – these 'deaths of despair' – drags down the average life expectancy. And since it's an annual estimate, it's highly sensitive to sudden changes in premature mortality (dying young instead of old). To illustrate how time-sensitive life expectancy is as a statistic, in a single year of the COVID pandemic, life expectancy in the US was estimated to have fallen by 1.8 years.

Most of this book is about personal lifespan (and healthy lifespan at that) rather than the blunt average of population life expectancy.

A spot of history with some surprises: In 1840, Swedish women were the world's longest-lived people with a life expectancy of around 46 years. At the time of writing, it's Japanese women at 87 years. Since 1840, life expectancy has increased by three months a year. But until fairly recently that's not been due to old people dying older. The reason for increased life expectancy in the 19th and first half of the 20th centuries was that fewer mothers, babies, children and young people died, due to advances in obstetrics, antisepsis, infectious diseases and immunisation. In fact, demographers – people who study population patterns – say that they still don't fully understand all the reasons for this boom in living longer. But here's a statistic that didn't change. If you were 50 years old in 1890, your chances of getting to, say, 70 were exactly the same as a 50-year-old's in 1950, two world wars later. Yet life expectancy had shot through the roof because kids and young mothers were surviving. What's changed since 1950 is how long you can expect to live when you're 50 years old, 60 years old and even 80 years old. By 1950 in rich nations we'd done pretty well at saving young lives. What happened then was that middle-aged people stopped dying, or at least were much less likely to. The reasons are still not entirely clear but stopping smoking, reducing blood pressure and cholesterol, and some medical interventions have made a lot of difference.

Knowing and not knowing: In the 19th and early 20th centuries and today still in disadvantaged and First Nations communities, people lived and live with huge uncertainty about what age they might die. These days, there's much more certainty if you're in a reasonably well-off postcode that, unless you're very unlucky, you're going to die in your late 80s or possibly 90s. My mum and dad in Glasgow were the unhealthiest people you can imagine yet even they lived until their 90s thanks to modern medicine.

In the 21st century we've pretty much maxed out the benefits at age 50 and the increased lifespan to be gained has shifted to age 75 or 80.

The statistics are dramatic when you compare today's chances of dying to 50 years ago.

If you're 50 years old today, your chances of dying at that age are the equivalent of someone who was in their late 30s or early 40s during the 1960s.

If you're 80 today, your chances of dying at that age are the equivalent of someone in their late 60s or early 70s fifty years ago.

If you're 90 years of age today, your chances of dying at that age are the equivalent of someone 50 years ago who was in their early 80s.

Put another way, in 1950, the risk of death in the following 12 months for an 85-year-old woman in Sweden was 17 per cent. Today it's 7 per cent. The size of reductions have been similar for men and even people aged over 90.

The age of onset of dementia is being delayed by two to four years every decade, and deaths from heart attacks and strokes declined by 2–3 per cent per annum for many years, but that stopped in the US in 2010 and a few years later in Australia and now there are signs that deaths from cardiovascular disease are rising again. This may be due to the increasing prevalence of obesity and declines in physical activity in some populations.

So it's fragile.

There's a lot of lifespan inequality in the United States and too many people are dying young from the effects of economic inequality, postcode disadvantage and despair resulting in gun violence, preventable injuries, poor maternal and child outcomes, coronary heart disease, obesity, smoking, opioid deaths, other drug and alcohol deaths, and self-harm due to depression and distress. In Australia, life expectancy gains seem to have stalled largely due to premature deaths from obesity related diseases and also mental health issues. The scale of COVID-19 deaths in many nations will show up in life expectancy reverses and that's on top of obesity and smoking as causes of premature deaths.

Let's focus, though, on us as individuals and our lifespan.

Is there a limit to lifespan? Another way of putting this is whether there's a 'natural' age at death for human beings.

This argument can either depress you or fill you with hope depending on who you believe. I personally choose the hope pathway, otherwise I wouldn't have bothered writing this book, but I'll lay out the arguments and evidence for you.

The first thing to say is that whichever side scientists fall on this argument, they all agree on one thing. Economic and social inequality is the strongest fundamental determinant of a shortened life and healthspan because, as I've said again and again, socioeconomic variables predict death at an early age. The scientific debate is about what happens *after* you've removed that inequality and the environmental factors and health consequences that go with it. Is the biology immutable?

The proponents for there being a limit to lifespan and that we're close to it in many countries, say that when you study non-human primates and human populations going back hundreds of years, there is evidence that once you eliminate the statistical effect of deaths before adulthood, then biological ageing takes over and in most species that appears to occur at a fixed rate. The evidence is powerful and comes from really good researchers who've looked in depth at 39 datasets including wild and captive primates, human populations going back to the 16th century and some hunter-gatherers.

There are three main implications from what they're saying. First, as I just said, that when you subtract avoidable deaths and leave non-human and human primates to age naturally, ageing occurs at a set pace. That leads to a second conclusion, which is that it's going to be hard to put the brakes on ageing much less reverse it because you'll be fighting a pre-programmed process. The third and last implication is that this pre-programmed rate of natural ageing means there's a pre-programmed age at death. Some of the people on this side of the fence say that the absolute maximum lifespan of humans is around 115 years.

Whoever wrote Ecclesiastes maybe knew a thing or two:

> To every thing there is a season,
> and a time to every purpose under the heaven:
> A time to be born, a time to die …

However, it may not be immutable or necessarily predetermined. The folk singer Pete Seeger turned this biblical verse into a huge hit as an anti-war song, 'Turn, Turn, Turn'. His adaptation to add words about there being a time for peace, and the vow that it was not too late for peace, made a call against the inevitability of war.

There is actually common ground between the two sides of this argument. Those who believe ageing is not immutable, and that we're not showing any signs of reaching a lifespan limit, accept that once you survive through childhood and middle age, we do all tend to die around a similar age. That superficially sounds like there is a biologically predetermined rate of ageing. They also accept the maths, that if you lengthen lifespan at old age, you don't do much for the population's life expectancy, since you won't have added on as many years as you do by saving the life of a 5-year-old or even a 50-year-old. But what they do argue – and one of the leaders of this pack has been Professor James Vaupel of Duke University, the Max Planck Institute and the Danish Institute for Advanced Study – is that there is an 'advancing front of old age survival'. So these days, deaths in old age cluster around the late 80s and early 90s, whereas 50 years ago that cluster would have been 10 or

15 years earlier. That's got very little to do with life expectancy and everything to do with lifespan.

So how do you reconcile the powerful biological evidence of a fixed rate of ageing with this advancing front of old-age survival? It's not entirely clear but it's likely the explanation is that humans exposed to similar environments tend to age at the same rate, but that rate adapts to how we live. So if we stop smoking, don't put on too much weight, get a decent education when we're younger, inhale cleaner air and eat a healthier diet, then as a species we slow down ageing or at the very least the diseases of ageing which carry us off. But because we have similar biological make-up, every generation ends up dying together – just later and later.

Earlier I quoted the chances of dying at certain ages today compared to 50 years ago and Vaupel and his colleagues argue this frontier of ageing keeps getting pushed out and that the evidence for a lifespan limit of 115 is very thin. And change can happen quite quickly. Vaupel – who founded an institute of ageing in Germany – argues that after German Reunification death rates in the over 65s in East Germany quite rapidly fell to the same levels as the non-communist West Germany, suggesting the better social and medical infrastructure made a difference.

To paraphrase Jonathan Swift, we all want to live long but none of us want to get old, and the evidence goes backwards and forwards on whether we are actually living these extra years in pretty good shape. We still get sick and frail a few years before we die but those few years are occurring at older and older ages. It's called 'compression of morbidity'. The Global Burden of Disease Study, which for decades has been looking at years lost to premature death and disability, has found that while we are living longer we do accumulate disabilities in those extra years. The question is, how disabling are those disabilities? We might be living with heart disease on medication but don't notice it that much. We might have a stiff, arthritic knee but do well with exercise and quadriceps strengthening. You might have had breast cancer but new medications are prolonging your life, and there's pretty good evidence from some countries that dementia is occurring at older ages.

At the time of writing, the longest-lived person has been Mme Jeanne Calment, who died at age 122 in France. Vaupel predicts it won't be long before that record is broken.

Rejuvenation is a thing

#youngblood
#notallbullshit

Quick take: Sympathetic magic is probably ingrained in our genes. It goes back for tens of thousands of years and assumes we can absorb the properties of animals or other humans by variously sacrificing them, drawing them on the walls of caves or eating them. In the 21st century there are companies which will take thousands of dollars from you to infuse you with young blood to help you live younger longer. It appeals enormously to the magical beliefs we've evolved with but interestingly there is something to it, although it's not necessarily what these entrepreneurs are selling.

Parabiosis goes back to the 19th century. It's where you surgically attach two animals – usually mice – and watch what happens, especially if one mouse is old and the other young. Parabiosis has made a comeback among researchers, especially those interested in ageing. When you do this joining up, the old mouse rejuvenates, especially its liver, brain and muscles, and lives longer. The trouble with parabiosis is that it's a profound mingling of the two animals and the effects could be due to the young mouse's organs doing the work for the old codger it's stitched to. That led a group of researchers in California to develop a technique where the mice only share their blood. When that happens the story is altogether different and has shifted the focus away from searching for the factors in young bodies that make them young.

When an old and a young mouse just share their blood, the old mouse does get a bit younger but not much. The impact – cruelly – is on the youngster who starts to age quite rapidly. They experience less nerve regeneration in the hippocampus, which is essential for memory and thinking, and display reduced learning and agility and reduced liver regeneration. In other words, it looks as though there are substances in old blood which cause ageing and if you could find them and block their activity, then you might have a return route to youth. One such factor may be a chemical messenger, TGF-beta, which increases with age and sets off a cascade of pathways that may or may not be related to the ageing process. The same group of researchers who developed the blood sharing technique blocked one of these pathways, ALK5, using a low dose of an ALK5 inhibitor for a short time. They used a short burst of a low dose to avoid the body's standard stubbornness and resistance to change – the homeostatic adaptation that I talked about earlier.

Oxytocin: The researchers also added oxytocin, a hormone produced in the brain and production of which falls with age. Oxytocin is used medically to induce labour but has all kinds of roles in the body. For example, it's being trialled as a medication for anxiety and depression and developmental issues such as autism. Oxytocin is thought to play a role in the homeostatic disruption of ageing. It is known to increase muscle regeneration, has few side effects and could be given in a nose spray.

In this experiment (yes, in mice) they found increased nerve growth in the hippocampus, reduced inflammation in the brain, increased muscle and liver regeneration, and improved cognitive performance. They also found evidence of lower levels of cellular senescence – old cells which can cause havoc and increase the rate of ageing (see Putting Out the Garbage).

A word of warning about what look like anti-ageing factors – they might not work the way studies suggest they might. A messenger called GDF11 is an example. GDF11 is a relative of TGF-beta and there's evidence that it increases nerve growth and blood supply, but also disturbing evidence to the contrary that GDF11 may actually kill brain cells. There are too many small, poorly designed studies in animals which may have no relevance to humans or be distorted by how much is given how often.

Stem cells: Some people still think that what's going to work is transfusing young blood into old people, assuming there are factors in blood from a young person that can rejuvenate. While there's a tiny amount of evidence for plasma transfusions from young donors in people with Alzheimer's disease, the results from various studies are not overly optimistic. Plasma, by the way, is blood without the red and white blood cells and there are concerns that young blood or plasma could either overactivate tissues, creating a cancer risk, or cause 'parabiotic disease' which may be a form of tissue rejection.

Other people have said that what older people need is young stem cells. There are two big picture ageing processes: the passing of time which allows the steady accumulation of aged (senescent) cells which I'll cover later; and cell replication and renewal which is partly what we're talking about here – and a little later, when I talk about telomeres.

So let's look at stem cells and cell replication. Some researchers argue that rejuvenation is when you shift the balance in the body from tissue *degeneration* to *regeneration and repair*. Stem cells are the source of tissue regeneration and repair. They're the parent cells which can either become any tissue at all (pluripotent) or are more specifically programmed to turn into cells like heart, muscle and brain. Either way, stem cells seem to thin out as we age and lose their ability to repair and regenerate, which means we become weaker, less resilient and descend into frailty. Stem cells are sensitive to inflammation damage and what are called 'epigenetic changes', where the shape and function of genes are changed. That's the DNA methylation I mentioned earlier. One promising avenue of anti-ageing research is into substances called 'Yamanaka factors', named after the Nobel-Prize-winning scientist who discovered how to create pluripotent stem cells.

Trouble is that when you infuse young stem cells into an older animal, they rapidly start looking like old stem cells. It turns out that the problem of ageing stem cells isn't so much in the cells themselves but in the surrounding tissues where they live. If they end up in old tissues, it's like landing in residential aged care where if you're there long enough you're institutionalised to start behaving like the other residents. Sometimes the young stem cells even die, presumably from the shock of the new environment. In technical-speak, the age of stem cells is determined by the age of their 'niche'. The implication is that there's no point in transplanting stem cells. You've got to rejuvenate the environment of the ones you have already. That's what parabiosis seems to do. But stitching yourself to a younger person isn't hugely practical and when you share blood, it's the younger person who changes (for the worse).

Here's an experiment that'll do your head in.

The same research group in California took old mice and diluted their blood by half with saline and albumin. In other words, they didn't infuse young blood. They just diluted old blood by half. They called it 'neutral age blood exchange'. Lo and behold they got better rejuvenation than with parabiosis, without the risks. There was increased muscle repair, increased nerve regeneration in the hippocampus, and reduced fat and scarring in the liver. They didn't alter the total amount of albumin in the body, so it wasn't the albumin that had the effect. What they think was going on was that the ageing factors in old blood were diluted and that freed up rejuvenation processes. The dilution made old tissues young, in theory, by allowing stem cells to do their job again. In medicine there's a technology that does a similar kind of dilution. It's called 'therapeutic plasma exchange' or TPE. The researchers tried it in four people aged 65–70 (in other words, a tiny study) and found evidence of increased muscle regeneration and repair. If this effect is real, then it has the advantage of cutting across a variety of organs and tissues and ageing pathways, which again – in theory – could avoid allowing the body to adapt and fight against the new homeostasis.

High intensity aerobic exercise, by the way, has a similar effect by increasing lean body mass, improving insulin sensitivity, increasing muscle protein and enhancing mitochondrial function. Exercise plus metformin (see Which Pill and Why?) improves mitochondrial function in the brains (of animals).

Anyway, back to therapeutic plasma exchange because the tantalising prospect is that it might be useful in reversing age-related diseases like Alzheimer's. A small trial in people with Alzheimer's disease did show promise but that's a long way from launching it as a therapy, especially as TPE does have complications, although most are mild when carried out in experienced units.

*

The next sections look at what we as individuals might do to break away from the pack and live younger even longer.

A word of warning, though: there's quite a lot that can come along and seriously stuff this up. These include warfare, more and worse pandemics, environmental degradation, extreme temperatures, worsening pollution, economic collapse, and no end to an obesity pandemic driven by profit in the globalised food industry. #justsaying

PART 2

Eating – not fasting – holds the secret

#wearentmice
#wearentfruitflies
#wecertainlyarentworms

Small bite: Here's the thing you've got to watch out for – and it's obvious when you think about it. If someone wakes up one morning with a brilliant idea that will make us live to 120 in great shape, you're going to be a distant memory before they find out whether it works or not. And the challenge of proof gets harder as we live longer. In other words, you'll have to hang on until people reach 120 before you know. The worst area of all is nutrition because all the time you've got people telling you what you should eat and how, and experimenting with your diet in a way that you'd never let them if they were pushing a drug. I'll give you the punchline now. At the current stage of research and knowledge about slowing ageing, there's one intervention that appears to work across all species, starting with worms and fruit flies, then into mice and non-human primates, with positive signals in humans. In fact, it's the gold standard against which all other anti-ageing interventions are measured. What I'm blathering on about is dietary restriction – largely meaning calorie restriction while maintaining healthy nutrition. It's been studied since at least 1917 but there are lots of nuances, including whether the secret in the sauce is calories, protein or even when and how much you eat across the day. The starting point, though, is what you eat freely when the guilt monkey is not on your back. It's called 'ad libitum feeding'.

Ad libitum is the curse on my head and my visceral fat. It's eating how much and how often you like and that's a problem for me because I have a very poorly functioning off-switch. Actually, now that I think about it, my off-switch is pretty much non-functioning. In a restaurant it starts with the menu. Regardless of the cost of the dishes, I over-order and, having over-ordered, when the food comes, it nonetheless all gets eaten. If I'm out with fellow Jews or almost anyone from an ethnic minority, they see this as normal behaviour. Catholics are also pretty relaxed as a group but Protestants can't cope. At a buffet, it usually means hovering near the buffet table while trying to have deep and meaningful conversations with half my brain preoccupied by the nearby food. In my home, it means trying to leave the fridge empty so there's no reason to visit it. One of my many most embarrassing lifetime moments occurred when I was being taken by a real estate agent to look at a house for sale. She let me wander around. Some time clearly went by so she came to find me … I'd opened the fridge in a complete stranger's house and was gazing into it in a trance-like state. She didn't say anything. She had no need to. I quietly closed the fridge, having made a mental note to try the brand of pickled cucumbers they had, and moved off to inspect the sink. How much of this is genetic I know not, but I have noticed that when one of my daughters visits, she heads straight to the fridge and is visibly disappointed if it's in one of its empty phases.

I tell you this for no other reason than to explain that ad libitum is the state which is the comparator when animals or indeed humans are put on dietary restriction to see what it does to lifespan or the factors which might perpetuate your youth for as long as possible.

There's a long list of lab animals and organisms who've been subjected to dietary restriction and have been reported to live longer. In rising order of biological complexity, they include yeast, worms, fruit flies, houseflies, mice, rats and monkeys. Dietary restriction is really calorie restriction, usually 10–50 per cent below what the animal would eat if left to it (ad libitum). In these experiments the calorie-restricted diets are carefully designed to avoid malnutrition. But there is a sweet spot because when dietary restriction is too severe, animals die sooner.

In rhesus monkeys, dietary restriction has been shown to reduce obesity (well, you'd hope so), cancer, brain degeneration, frailty and diabetes; seems to make their genes less likely to mutate; reduces inflammation (inflammation is probably one of the causes of ageing); and improves how effective insulin is at reducing blood sugar (insulin sensitivity). Dietary-restricted monkeys (30 per cent below ad libitum) have half the chances of dying at any age and have a bio-age that's seven years younger than non-restricted monkeys of the same chronological age. This is not simply explained by less heart disease, diabetes and cancer. The animals are physiologically younger – their 'intrinsic ageing' is slowed down. For example, they are less likely to experience age-related hearing loss, which is thought to be due to ageing of the hearing mechanism. Similarly they experience less sarcopaenia – the loss of muscles due to the ageing process.

Most of this research has been in laboratories in animals bred for experimentation. The extent to which an animal will respond to dietary restriction seems to have a genetic basis. In other words, the contribution of genes to how long an animal lives is around 30 per cent if they're eating an ad libitum diet. In animals who respond to dietary restriction by living longer, the contribution of genes is nearly 55 per cent. So, different breeds of animals respond in different ways and scientists often deliberately select responsive breeds. Another source of confusion is that ad libitum is not always what it seems. Well-meaning researchers have given the control animals a healthy diet and that might narrow the added benefit of dietary restriction, since a healthy diet by itself makes you live longer in good health.

Of course, we aren't rats or mice, so monkeys have been of great interest because non-human primates are closer genetically to us. There have been two long-term studies of dietary restriction in monkeys and they came up with different results. They didn't primarily look at lifespan, more at *how* they survived. In a study published in 2009, 80 per cent of restricted monkeys survived to old age compared to 50 per cent on ad libitum diets. The reason seemed to be due to less cancer, diabetes and heart disease. Another monkey study reported in 2012 failed to show the same effect, but when both studies were re-analysed, the conclusion was that the calorie-restricted monkeys in the second study actually did do better. In fact, six out of 20 of the original monkeys lived to over 40 years old, which is remarkable since other studies have found that 40 is the outer limit of maximum lifespan in normal monkeys. The other debate was whether dietary restriction had to start in childhood to get the benefit and the review concluded it worked if you started in adulthood.

The bottom line is that dietary restriction in animals does seem to increase lifespan and with added healthy years (healthspan).

So what about humans? Well, as I said before, you've got to wait a heck of a long time to get an answer but there are some signs. A small, two-year trial put healthy, non-obese young to middle-aged adults on a 12 per cent reduced calorie diet. They lost 10 per cent of their body weight and had lower LDL (bad cholesterol) levels, lower blood pressure, and lower levels of inflammation as measured by a test called 'C reactive protein (CRP)' and that reduction seemed to be independent of the weight loss. The researchers credited the calorie restriction and claimed that these measures indicated that if the benefits persisted, those people would likely have longer lives in good health. It makes for a powerful story which is reinforced by how central dietary restriction has become to understanding what happens at the molecular level to the cascade of chemical reactions at the core of ageing. In other words, in the 'test tube' the effects of dietary restriction have become the benchmark when they've been looking for anti-ageing pills or supplements.

Dietary restriction reduces oxidative stress – biological rusting – but that doesn't mean you can get out of eating less by swallowing antioxidant supplements, which don't seem to prevent anything very much apart from the beneficial effects of exercise. That's probably because they're not natural and are taken in vastly higher doses than you get in cooked food which contains thousands of compounds that work with each other.

What makes the difference?

Is it calories? Is it protein? Is it how much you eat at what time of day? What about fasting? Remember, most of what I'm about to describe comes from experiments in animals that are often genetically engineered to exaggerate some aspect of the ageing process or metabolism. There are too few good studies in humans so far.

Protein

There's a signal from research that protein matters in dietary restriction but at the moment the evidence is conflicting and confusing. There is some evidence that reducing protein intake reduces body fat, and, conversely, eating a reduced-calorie diet with high protein content may lower the benefits of dietary restriction. Some research suggests that specific amino acids (the building blocks of proteins) may increase or slow ageing.

Be very careful about believing any of that at this stage. Protein intake is important to prevent muscle wasting and keep your immune system running well, so don't mess with it too much.

Meal timing?

While I'm talking about protein, since one of its many purposes is to maintain and build muscle, research in humans points to getting the best muscle synthesis by spreading your protein intake evenly through the day. What most of us do, though, is load most of our protein into dinner. One study in healthy men and women in their 30s directly compared the normal pattern of protein intake, which is skewed to dinner, to evenly spread intake throughout the day and found the muscle synthesis rate was 25 per cent higher in the 'evenly spread' group. Another study on protein intake following resistance exercise in healthy men confirmed that evenly spread protein intake was best for muscle synthesis. A very significant part of successfully living younger longer is having strong muscles and avoiding the muscle wasting that accompanies ageing (sarcopaenia). That leads to frailty which leads to premature death.

Time-restricted eating (e.g. the 16:8)

This is about eating early or late with fasting in between. One of the most popular forms of time-restricted eating is only eating between 12 p.m. and 8 p.m. and fasting from then until midday the next day. Most of the studies have been small and badly designed. One of the better ones took people who were mostly in their 40s and were overweight or obese. The comparator to 16:8 was three meals a day. They all lost weight but there was no difference between the overnight fasting group and the three-meals-a-day group, nor were there any greater metabolic benefits. One of the troubling findings in this trial was that in the time-restricted eating group, 65 per cent of their weight loss was from losing lean muscle mass. That compares to 20–40 per cent in other weight loss regimes. It would be very unfortunate if 16:8 eating speeded up the path to sarcopaenia. Early eating has also been trialled with mixed results. A study of men with pre-diabetes who ate early in the day and fasted from the afternoon to breakfast found that their blood fats (cholesterol and triglycerides) went up, which probably reinforces that it's not enough to restrict your diet, you've got to pay attention to what you're eating. And if you aren't confused enough, a study of women with polycystic ovary syndrome (PCOS), which involves being overweight or obese, having fertility issues and sometimes masculinisation, found that biasing calorie intake to breakfast and early in the day improved insulin sensitivity, increased weight loss and reduced testosterone levels.

Point being that this is complex stuff and doesn't lend itself to simple solutions. Professor Luigi Fontana, a world authority on dietary restriction, argues strongly that what you eat in dietary restriction must be close to the Mediterranean diet to ensure optimal nutritional intake and that this should be accompanied by moderately intense exercise to ensure your metabolic rate – your background calorie burn – doesn't adapt to the calorie restriction by turning down the dial. Exercise keeps it up.

Circadian (body clock) rhythms

Growing evidence suggests that your body clocks – there are many of them – have a significant influence on how quickly you age and your risk of metabolic and brain issues like dementia. (I write much more about circadian rhythm and staying young in Does the Mind Matter?) In relation to eating and fasting, it's a two-edged sword. Playing around with your eating times can mess up your circadian rhythm, with unknown consequences. On the other hand, deliberately adjusting eating times may help get a disrupted body clock system back into sync and protect against ageing processes. It's another thing to think about when a health guru offers you a simple diet solution. Also, when your clock is 'out' it can drive overeating and the development of obesity.

What about fasting?

Fasting as a solution for weight loss and avoiding other ills such as diabetes has sold millions of books over the last few years. Let me remind you, however, of the H.L. Mencken quote at the beginning of this book. Paraphrased, it's that for every complicated problem there's a clear and simple solution ... which is usually wrong. I'd change 'wrong' to 'oversold compared to the evidence' for many of the simple answers offered in diet books.

A lot of the evidence on the effects of fasting comes from animal studies, particularly in mice and rats, and there are lots of issues translating what happens in small mammals to large ones like humans. First of all, we humans are much more able to tolerate fasting than rodents, which are metabolically stressed more easily than we are. The effects of fasting in rodents are also very specific to the genetic strain of mouse or rat being used. For example, in animal experiments of fasting, cancer protection does not always occur. Intermittent fasting in rodents can raise brain-derived neurotrophic factor (BDNF), which is linked to nerve growth and improvements in learning and memory. In studies of intermittent fasting in middle-aged humans, though, BDNF levels have been shown to decrease. It's not that there's no evidence of benefit in human fasting, it's just that it's inconsistent and sometimes dependent on whether you're obese.

But what if you're not obese and you want to live longer younger, does intermittent fasting extend your years? Most of the research has been into short-lived animals like mice and fruit flies (*Drosophila*) and even then the scientific literature is a bit of a minefield. One study of intermittent fasting in fruit flies, where they were fasted for five days and fed for two (kind of the opposite of the 5:2 diet), actually *reduced* their lifespan unless it was given in the fruit flies' 'childhood' and middle age (a month in a *Drosophila*'s life). This fasting diet increased lifespan by around 10 per cent if given in early life and seemed to be via stress adaptation and gut health. I'm stating the bleeding obvious here, that we're not fruit flies and you wouldn't consider in a million years starving your young child or teenager, five days in every seven. Doesn't seem to work well in Sub-Saharan Africa or war-torn refugee camps. However, what research like this does show – again – is that calorie intake and longevity are linked.

Yeast responds to the yeast equivalent of fasting by becoming more stress resistant and living longer. Mice given a very low calorie diet (aimed at mimicking fasting) for four days every two weeks, followed by eating what they liked, showed improvements in brain function, brain cell growth (neurogenesis), tummy fat, bone density and lowered cancer risk which was associated with these mice living longer on average – although the maximum lifespan wasn't affected. A small preliminary trial from the same research group of a five day a month, plant-based, very low calorie diet for three cycles showed benefits in terms of inflammation, blood sugar control, reducing a cancer-related hormone called 'insulin-like growth factor', and signs that cellular regeneration might have been occurring. The assumption was that if larger studies bore that out, you'd have to think that this would eventually extend human lives too, in good shape. This fits with the Greek paradox that I wrote about in my previous book, *So You Think You Know What's Good For You?* (See Intermittent Frugality below.)

The very low calorie diet?

In the past few years, very low calorie diets – say, 800 calories a day – have become popular for losing weight if you're obese, particularly if the diet is low in carbs and therefore ketogenic. The evidence suggests that if you're obese and are losing control of your blood sugar and heading for diabetes, then this kind of diet does work – at least for a while – but you should be supervised and have it planned so you're getting the right intake of nutrients and protein to preserve your muscle mass and avoid serious deficiencies. A well-designed diet of 500–800 calories a day seems to be better than a standard low calorie diet at reducing waist circumference, BMI, blood fats (especially triglycerides), blood pressure and insulin levels, and improving blood sugar control. For the technically minded, the carbs should be less than 50 g a day, the protein intake should be 1–1.5 g per kilogram of your ideal weight, and the fat content should be about 15–30 g per day.

All that should add up to extra years of life in good shape if you start off from the disadvantage of being obese but no-one knows for sure. It's certainly not a lifelong dietary pattern.

Intermittent frugality (vegan fasting)

#isthisthenewthing

Accept Greeks bearing gifts: The Trojan Horse has all sorts of stuff inside for the long-lived lifestyle.

According to research at Deakin University, the second-longest-lived people in the world are first generation Greek Australians. They've been best studied in Melbourne, which is said to be the third-largest Greek city in the world after Thessaloniki. These Greek migrants even live longer than the brothers and sisters they left behind in Greece. The first assumption you make when you hear this is that it's all due to the Mediterranean diet and it's true that the Med diet has something to do with it. However, early research into this group showed that when they first arrived in Melbourne, they did not necessarily follow their traditional diet. They loved the abundance of red meat in Australia and went a bit nuts on it. In time, though, they did return to more traditional eating, which in the style of the Greek Islands is high in plant-based foods, beans and lentils, fish and fowl for protein, olive oil for fat, and not much red meat.

But that's only part of the story.

For a start, they pride themselves on using fresh ingredients. They have a backyard or allotment where they grow their own herbs and vegetables – which means both getting some exercise and having produce that has retained high levels of potential anti-ageing compounds.

Then it's how they cook because cuisine counts for a lot. Cooking in the Mediterranean style creates anti-ageing compounds with an intensity that you could never replicate in bottled supplements in your local chemist. Red vegetables like tomatoes and capsicum when chopped and cooked in extra virgin olive oil produce potent antioxidants. When you cook onions, garlic, herbs and tomatoes in extra virgin olive oil, the same kind of chemical magic occurs. It turns out that cooking can make food even healthier than eating it raw.

That's not always the case, though. Some food traditions are pretty unhealthy, like the Jewish/Scottish cuisine I grew up with – fries twice a day, vegetables cooked to a mush, and Eastern European dishes hotching with red meat, carbs and saturated fat. When you went out for a meal, it wasn't much better. Glasgow was, and still is, an epicentre of Indian cuisine and it so happens that India vies with Glasgow for having the highest rate of coronary heart disease in the world. To give you some idea of how entrenched Indian food is in Glasgow, a few years ago on a visit, I went with my brothers to a popular Indian restaurant. The elderly Indian waiters spoke with strong Glaswegian accents which had not a trace of South Asia. The menu was so large it had a contents page with a section called 'Scottish Favourites'. *Hello,* I thought, *this is for people who inexplicably don't like Indian food and will have stuff like haggis and fish and chips.* Nope. The Scottish Favourites page was where they put boring old dishes like rogan josh, beef vindaloo and lamb madras, no doubt all laden with ghee but

77

much loved by Scottish university students looking for a cheap, flavoursome meal.

I digress. Back to Melbourne and Greek Australians, because the other part of their cooking style is that they do it slowly. Slow cooking minimises burning and browning (caramelisation), and that brown stuff on the surface of foods can contain pro-ageing compounds called 'advanced glycation end products' or AGEs (more about these later in the book).

Next, they tend to eat with family and friends. Social support is an important element of living longer younger.

And finally, many Greek Australians follow the traditions of the Greek Orthodox Church, one of which is having about 100 fast days a year. Not intermittent fasting type fasts. More like vegan fasts where they don't eat animal protein for a day.

Frugal, green days. Maybe that's more sustainable in the long run.

The long-life kitchen chemistry set

#whatscookin
#teamsport

Come in from the barbie, guys: The kitchen is where you cook up extra healthy years. The ingredients you use, their freshness, what you put with what at what temperature, all make a difference. The aim is reducing harmful stuff on the plate and enhancing the good things.

I spent my years at medical school in a caravan. I know. I know. Luxury. It was the height of the oil boom in the North East of Scotland with soaring rents, and a classmate and I reckoned we'd save money if we bought a residential caravan and set ourselves up in that. We found one right across from the beach in the countryside just outside of town. Fourteen miles of unbroken, undisturbed silver sands. And that's where we lived. Now before you get images of California dreaming, I might remind you that this was the North East of Scotland. The lapping waves were the North Sea and the winds came uninterrupted from northern Europe and Russia. In the six years I lived in that caravan, I went into the sea once – on a warm summer's day (again, note the temperature was the equivalent of what I now know is a cold winter's day in Sydney) – and stayed in the water for a languorous 15 seconds. Cold doesn't come close to describing life in that caravan. There were two bedrooms – a single and a double – and we switched every term, although since my caravan mate was a good-looking Jamaican who played tight head prop for Scottish Universities, he had more need of the double bedroom than me. Anyway, the point of this story is not about student sex in small spaces, it's to tell you that this is where I learned to cook. Sunday nights in our caravan were famous because we had people drive out to us for dinner. Our lounge room was the size of a small bathroom, yet we managed to squeeze in whoever would turn up. Having no money, meat was a small part of any dish, and we ranged from West Indian to Indian to what we'd now know as Mediterranean. When I arrived in Australia, I could actually make quite complex dishes but I had no idea how to cook a steak. In fact, I still don't. While that's embarrassing to admit, it turns out not necessarily to be a bad thing.

Any good chef will tell you that cooking is chemistry and they know the effect they'll achieve when they put in a herb, increase temperature, add or subtract salt, or whatever. Most restaurant chefs, though, are going for taste and impact and if it's a little bit unhealthy what the heck, it's only one meal and you want to make it memorable. However, not one of these chefs would be the slightest bit surprised by what's going on in the pot or the baking dish at a molecular level. This isn't to detract from the romance and gestalt of cooking and eating because they do matter, but let's dwell on what's happening beneath the surface.

When the chemistry's right in the pot, it produces substances which keep us young. They're called bioactives. I'll come back to the recipe for bioactives in a minute.

You see, while we don't know as much as you'd think about what ages us, the process goes something like this. We rust from the inside out. We need oxygen to live but when oxygen is metabolised it throws off highly dangerous oxygen atoms which combine with other chemicals, creating very unstable molecules called 'free radicals'. In their search for stability, free radicals stick to tissue anywhere in our bodies and when they do they cause some damage – just the way oxygen does when it clings to unprotected iron. It's called 'oxidation' and the effect is oxidative stress. The path to living younger longer is paved with reducing oxidative stress. When you look at large groups of people, those with low levels of natural antioxidants like lycopene and carotenoids tend to be more likely to die young instead of old and have higher than average rates of heart disease and memory and thinking problems.

There's a multibillion-dollar global industry which sells this idea in a bottle. They flog you antioxidant supplements which they claim reduce oxidative stress. Trouble is that they don't work. Large studies (sadly) show no benefit in terms of preventing common diseases of ageing such as heart attacks and dementia. You're on much safer ground betting your future on what's on your cooker (sorry, stove) and on your plate. And where do these antioxidants come from? Well, significantly from red, orange and purple vegetables, especially when they're cooked in extra virgin olive oil.

It's doing a disservice to substances like flavonoids and carotenoids to call them antioxidants because they often do so much more than reduce oxidative stress. That's why I'd prefer to call them bioactives because they help communication inside cells and can make metabolism go more smoothly.

Inside our cells are tiny energy factories and communications centres called mitochondria. Like any power station, they produce pollution. That pollution is made up of pro-oxidants; substances like free radicals, which make us rust and progressively damage the mitochondria themselves and the tissues around them. One measure of ageing is having clapped-out mitochondria. For example, a feature of getting older is that your muscles weaken unless you work on them. It's called 'sarcopaenia'. Sarcopaenic muscles have clapped-out mitochondria. Interestingly, research at McMaster University in Ontario has shown that if someone with sarcopaenia weight trains, their mitochondria rejuvenate. It shows that ageing is not a one-way street.

Another example of the damage that can be done is atherosclerosis, the major cause of heart disease, where bad cholesterol (LDL) gets caught up in the side walls of our arteries, irritates the immune system and then thanks to the pro-oxidants in our blood, rusts the arteries, narrowing them and making them fragile so they're exposed to creating artery-blocking blood clots. The biggest pro-oxidant of all is tobacco smoke, which is why smokers have hugely increased risks of atherosclerosis, heart attacks, vascular dementia and stroke. Saturated fat and sunlight are also pro-oxidants.

By the way, you can't separate out one thing from another, these factors all work together – the bad actors and the good ones, the bad team and the good team. In the case of the pro-oxidants from smoking, they also make the platelets in your blood more sticky. Platelets are the first step in the creation of a blood clot, so while the bad team is stuffing up your arteries from the inside, they're preparing your blood for an easy clot when the atherosclerosis breaks through.

Back to antioxidants, or rather bioactives, because just as the bad guys work together, so do the good ones. It's a complex team sport that can't be replicated in a bottle. To continue the metaphor, team sports require intense communication between players on the field. These bioactives don't just counteract oxidants and biological rusting, they also pass messages and help cells and mitochondria communicate with each other. The body needs harmony. Cancer prevention, for example, relies on it. There's evidence that the signals cells need so they can die naturally come from mitochondria with help from bioactives. This is a process called 'apoptosis' and many, if not all, cancers are a failure of natural cell death which results in cells multiplying out of control.

Not all bioactives come from our food but even when they don't, they are influenced by what we eat. For example, some are produced by a healthy microbiome in the gut, especially one called butyrate, which is thought to be particularly potent at firing up a chemical process that slows ageing, protects the brain and preserves apoptosis.

So ... here's the recipe for your natural, staying young as long as possible, chemistry set.

Use red and reddish vegetables a lot. Chop them (that helps to release their bioactives) and cook slowly in extra virgin olive oil which has its own bioactives. Add onions and garlic and herbs, all of which make the chemistry more complex and fruitful. It may be important what order you do this, which is why sofrito is a good base to start with (onions, garlic, tomatoes and sometimes carrots cooked together at a moderate temperature). Australian research has shown that these culinary processes release far more bioactives than eating these foods raw. The cooking also makes them more available to the body; in other words, more likely to be absorbed. There's no point having bioactives if they can't be taken up by your body and used. Cooking enhances their utility, which includes making your platelets less sticky, thereby reducing the chances of developing blood clots to gum up your brain or heart.

The list of ingredients is long but the raw basics include tomatoes, carrots, red capsicum, beetroot and lots of fresh herbs, with watermelon for dessert. It also looks as though the cooking oil needs to be extra virgin olive oil. You don't seem to get the same effect from sunflower oil, for example.

Finally, the temperature at which you cook matters. Too high (e.g. on a barbecue) tends to burn or caramelise the food, and that brown stuff on the surface contains pro-oxidants. Slow cooking matters.

Goji berries, cider vinegar and magical thinking

#cidervinegarbythegallon

Quick swig: Look, if you're drinking gallons of apple cider vinegar each week to keep your youth, as they say, even if you don't live longer, it's so unpleasant you'll feel as though you are. Single food consumption in large amounts is not physiological. What I mean is that foods are supposed to be consumed together in normal quantities and usually exert their effects on our bodies in concert with other stuff in our diet, especially when cooked. When you take abnormally large amounts of a food, the dose is so high you're actually starting to use it as a drug even though you feel it's natural. Would you take a drug that hasn't been tested? Doubt it. So, have cider vinegar and goji berries by all means but don't obsess or gorge on them. Leave room for all the other foods and dishes that keep ageing at bay.

To hear me go on about them, you'd think I've got something against goji berries. I haven't. They're pretty fine berries chock-full of carotenoids – some of the antioxidants I was praising earlier – and they do appear to be highly bioavailable when they are – wait for it – mushed up with olive oil. Not sure how much you like your fruits with extra virgin olive oil. I'm writing this in the early morning, which is when my digestive system hovers between anorexia and nausea, so it sounds revolting. There is some evidence, though, that the kinds of antioxidants in goji berries might be good at protecting your retina – the cinema screen at the back of your eye on which we rely for our vision. So chomp away but don't bet the farm on goji berries as a single food solution.

Another single food that people are anecdotally consuming in large quantities is apple cider vinegar. The market is large and growing at around 12 per cent per annum. From animal studies it's been touted as helping with weight loss, improving blood sugar control, and polishing your blood fat profile – all measures that are reasonable proxies for living more years healthier. Sad to say, the apple cider vinegar industry has been promoting itself on rather flimsy evidence in humans. There are signs that it may do some of those things and few if any indications of harm. So if you just love your vinegar in the morning then swill away. If not, then money saved and probably little else lost.

Just one more example: flaxseed oil.

I have a fondness for flax. I wear linen whenever I can get away with that crushed look (which, as you know, starts three nanoseconds after buttoning up the shirt or putting on the jacket). My paternal grandmother was born in the Latvian town of Dvinsk – where the abstract painter Mark Rothko was also born a few years later – and her father made his living in the surrounding fields as a flax cutter. So flax is in my genes, I suppose. Flaxseed oil has become popular amongst humans while it's almost identical twin, linseed, has been used for animal feed for a lot longer. There are plenty of goodies in flaxseed such as plant-based omega 3 fatty acids, alpha-linolenic acid and polyphenols called lignans which make plant-based oestrogens (phytoestrogens). All of which, especially the polyunsaturated fats, should help to reduce the risk of coronary heart disease. The trouble is bioavailability – that is, being able to absorb and allow your body to use the goodies. A bit like the story of the Mediterranean diet and how cuisine and cooking ingredients count, flaxseed may be at its most useful when processed as an oil and perhaps mixed with other oils. The trouble is that the people touting flaxseed oil can overstep the evidence. For example, they assume because it has phytoestrogens that it'll be great for preventing prostate cancer when, sadly, there's very little evidence that plant-based oestrogens have much, if any, effect on the body. Again it comes down to whether you're using flaxseed oil as a drug to keep you young or as a substitute for other oils in your cooking and diet. If as a drug then there's almost no research of value in humans to support the marketed benefits although there's unlikely to be harm. If as an ingredient in cooking, then flaxseed oil might be a handy addition. The other potential problem is that the unsaturated fats in flaxseed can deteriorate over a few months, which is why some researchers argue it needs to be mixed into a stable oil emulsion.

I could go on with other examples of an excess of hope from using foods as drugs. I'd love to write you a book which tells you that the way to stay young is easy and my publisher would like it even more. However, while it's not that hard, you're still fighting pretty powerful biology, so staying young needs to be confronted from more than one angle and requires effort from the kitchen to the gym – and maybe, just maybe, the medicine cabinet.

Remember what we're fighting here is homeostasis, the body's balancing act; its survival mechanism trying to keep an even keel even when the boat might be firmly tilted towards ageing.

Think big when it comes to food

… because thinking small costs you money on stuff that literally goes down the drain and may not get you anywhere.

This is worth labouring briefly before we get to the next section because what follows is the small stuff; in other words, the hope that single substances can make you live longer in youthful shape. It may be true and it's filled with hope but don't forget the basics.

We've been filled with health anxieties – often by people who want to make money out of them. These fears are about all sorts of things: too little sleep, not drinking enough water, low carbs, high protein, paleo, the fact that we don't look like Brad Pitt or a Kardashian, which supplement should I be taking, etc etc.

The message – again – is: sweat the big stuff. Exercise as intensively as you're able or allowed to, as many days of the week as you can, including intentionally strengthening your muscles (see Outrunning the Clock and Get a Grip). And with your food – to paraphrase the food and science writer Michael Pollan – eat more plants, less meat and only stuff that your granny would recognise as food. And to paraphrase me: cook your food in moderate heat with fresh ingredients, lots of herbs, garlic and onions and red and orange vegetables, in extra virgin olive oil.

That's while you wait to see if a magic pill turns up that can keep you young as long as possible. The next part lists the main hopefuls at the moment. I'm sure there will be more in the future.

PART 3

Which pill and why?

#hopespringseternal

Quick swallow: You've got the message by now. You and I are not fruit flies, yeast cells or mice. If we were, there'd be little cancer and we'd live long, healthy lives because science has found stuff that works in the lab but fails in humans. Same goes for the millions if not billions of dollars that have been wasted in the wrong-headed search for a drug for Alzheimer's disease. Don't get me going about dementia researchers but the same thing applies to pharmaceuticals that might halt, slow or reverse ageing. Plenty of disappointments in humans but there are some green shoots of promise. We're just so much more complicated than wee animals that scurry around wheat silos.

If my grandparents were to come back today, they'd be amazed and amused. They were migrants from one cold, tough land (Russia) to another (Scotland), which although a struggle, allowed them to advance and make good lives for themselves and their children. They didn't like ageing. In fact, I remember my paternal grandmother – the one from Dvinsk who had a thick Eastern European accent all her life – telling me that the 'vorst ting vos' having a mind that still felt young but in a body that just couldn't keep up. Having said that, they kind of accepted it. My maternal grandfather would get up in the morning, make the fire (yes, with coal) then sit there in his vest making a terrible noise as he tried to clear his chest of a lifetime of smoking. He swore by hot water or Russian tea with lemon and a wee bit of sugar. And just to spoil the Russian romance, dentists will tell you that there's nothing more poisonous for your teeth than hot citrus with sugar. I'm rambling, but my point is that if my grandparents came back they'd be amazed at the rejection of ageing on the one hand and the relative youth of people who today are the same age that they were when they died of heart disease and cancer.

My grandparents, who left school at age 14, certainly hadn't read Dylan Thomas who, in 1947, was already headlong into self-destruction yet wrote that he raged at the 'dying of the light'.

Today's raging young old have generally worked hard to retain their youth but wouldn't it be great if a pill could save all that trouble, even if it wouldn't have saved Thomas from his alcoholism and smoking.

The scientists' playbook for developing an anti-ageing pill generally comes from what they know about the effects of calorie (or dietary) restriction on animals at a molecular level. Dietary restriction does a lot of things to our metabolism, but it's the effect on one particular enzyme which fires up some researchers into ageing. Enzymes are substances which help chemical reactions to take place. Molecular helpers, if you like. This one is called SIRT1 and when turned on in yeast, roundworms, fruit flies and perhaps some other organisms, it's associated with a longer lifespan. SIRT1 is linked to the rejuvenation of mitochondria, which are the powerhouses inside our cells; increased resistance to oxidative stress (biological rusting); improved cell survival and reduced inflammation. Animal studies have also suggested there's an important role for SIRT1 in protecting the brain and heart. This gets even more complicated, as you can imagine, but the core process that sits behind SIRT1 and which it relies upon, is a substance called NAD+.

NAD+ is involved in a lot of stuff inside our cells, from producing energy to cleaning up DNA to mopping up oxidative stress to helping genes communicate with the rest of the cell and much more. The activity of NAD+ declines with age and is also a target of anti-ageing researchers but most interest has been focused downstream on SIRT1.

Enter red wine and resveratrol.

Resveratrol – it might work

Resveratrol has been made famous by Professor David Sinclair, an expatriate Australian researcher based at Harvard University. David was one of the first to link the family of enzymes called sirtuins – to which SIRT1 belongs – to the complex process of ageing. Tantalisingly, resveratrol, which is found naturally in grapes, peanuts, berries and red wine to a varying extent, activates SIRT1 – which is biochemist-speak for saying it gets SIRT1 into action. As such, resveratrol – the existence of which has been known for decades – has been a handy laboratory tool to study SIRT1. However, using resveratrol to enhance SIRT1's activity could have profoundly beneficial effects on our bodies, from preventing cancer and heart disease to slowing the ageing process itself. In addition, resveratrol seems to have its own effects on other processes such as how cancer cells communicate with each other, the stickiness of platelets – the blood cells which trigger clots – strengthening heart muscle and improving blood sugar control.

When resveratrol has been tested in the test tube and animals, this promise has been borne out. The stumbling block, sadly – and hopefully temporarily – has been in humans. The studies have been small and poorly designed (for example, in some trials the participants who were on resveratrol knew they were on it rather than blinded), but found little harm apart from a signal about kidney damage in a trial of resveratrol in people with a blood cancer called multiple myeloma. A review of studies into resveratrol's effects on the brain found no changes to thinking and memory, mood, grey matter volume or blood pressure. A small but well-designed trial reported in 2020, of resveratrol in overweight and obese adults over a period of six months, found no improvements in how well insulin worked (insulin sensitivity), fat in the liver, body composition, blood pressure, quality of life, quality of sleep or physical performance. The only significant change was an improvement in blood sugar control averaged over three months.

There are several possible reasons for the failure of resveratrol so far. It has poor bioavailability, meaning it isn't easily absorbed and used by the body. Like many dietary substances, it seems to have different effects according to dose. In other words, it's possible that very low doses work differently from when you give resveratrol in more drug-like doses rather than as a micronutrient. This is not unusual and not a reason to give up on resveratrol just yet. Drug development often needs the work of medicinal chemists who can produce more potent and durable versions of natural compounds. The other possibility is that resveratrol might work best when taken with other pharmaceuticals which act on different parts of the ageing process. So the jury – as they say – is still out.

Metformin – it probably works

Metformin is causing a lot of interest because of its potential to be repurposed from what it is now – namely an effective diabetes medication which has the useful side effect of weight loss – into a medication that may prolong life with added years of health. Metformin is well studied in humans with diabetes and is cheap and relatively safe. The reasons why it's a candidate for an anti-ageing therapy stem mostly from animal and lab studies and what are called 'observational studies' of groups of people rather than properly designed experiments in randomised controlled trials.

In diabetes, metformin works by getting glucose out of the blood into cells where it's meant to be. It also reduces appetite and produces weight loss or at least minimises ongoing weight gain. Metformin was once believed – like resveratrol – to mimic the effects of dietary restriction but not many researchers still think that's true, although it does get involved in biochemical pathways that in lab animals appear to slow ageing and increase lifespan. Metformin may also have antioxidant properties that reduce oxidative stress and may also reduce the production of advanced glycation end products (AGEs), which increase oxidative stress and are thought to be one of the sources of the rapid ageing that's often seen in people with pre-diabetes or diabetes itself. The buzzword is 'geroprotective' and there are researchers who are convinced metformin is geroprotective while there are others who think the jury is still out. There is one narrow study in genetically distinct male mice which found a low dose of metformin extended a healthy lifespan while a higher dose was toxic. I can't find evidence of that study being replicated by others. There is also some evidence that metformin affects the gut microbiome, perhaps reducing the toxic effects of some bacteria or enhancing the beneficial effects of others.

The human evidence tends to come from observational studies – where groups of people are observed over a period of time and compared to each other or to similar people who don't have the disease being looked at. The gold standard, though, is the double-blind randomised controlled trial and there haven't been many of those, although some are in progress.

Observational studies can be fraught with biases. The first and most obvious is that you're usually dealing with people who have diabetes since that's what metformin is used for. Secondly, even comparing metformin use in diabetes is hard because people who are prescribed metformin are not necessarily the same as those who receive other medications. For instance, they are more likely to be overweight or obese and less likely to have kidney damage.

But anyway here's a sense of the human evidence for and against. A large review of observational studies found that people with diabetes taking metformin had a 7 per cent reduced risk of premature death compared to people without diabetes and a 6 per cent reduced incidence of cancer. In people with diabetes, metformin has been associated with a 25 per cent reduced risk of heart disease. Diabetes accelerates the risk of dementia along with ageing in general, and a memory and ageing study in Sydney, following more than 1000 people aged between 70 and 90 with no dementia at the start of the study, found that people with diabetes on metformin returned their risk of dementia to the same level as people who had no diabetes in the group. This was in comparison to people with diabetes in the study who were on other diabetes medications. So it wasn't just getting the blood sugar under control. There seemed to be an effect of metformin.

When you look at cancer studies across different cancer types, a general theme seems to emerge, which is that if you have diabetes and are on metformin you seem to do better on cancer treatment, but there is little evidence that metformin reduces the risk of developing cancer in the first place. To be fair, most people start metformin later in life when it may be too late to prevent cancer. Metformin can cause vitamin B12 and B6 deficiencies, which may be an issue. Having said that, the one cancer where there is some evidence of prevention is colorectal (bowel) cancer.

There are, however, some warning signals about metformin's effects on healthy ageing. A randomised trial in non-diabetic men and women aged 65 and older, to see whether metformin enhanced the beneficial effects of progressive resistance training, found instead a blunting effect of metformin on the muscle building effects of the exercise compared to placebo. A previous smaller study found reduced aerobic capacity.

There is no doubt that metformin is a great drug for people with diabetes. The issue which needs to be resolved is whether it benefits healthy people. There are ongoing trials of metformin in cancer, the prevention of frailty in the elderly and other studies which should hopefully sort out some of the answers rather than relying on assumptions made in the lab or potentially flawed observations in uncontrolled environments. Like resveratrol, it'd be great if metformin does fulfil its promise, but it may need the help of other anti-ageing compounds to straighten out the progressive and highly resistant tilt of homeostasis as we get older.

The Easter Island Effect

#doesrapkeepyouyoung

Soil sample: A substance discovered from the soil on Easter Island has helped to revolutionise thinking on how and why we age and how the speed at which we lose our youth is so wrapped up in the way we live and eat. The Easter Island discovery is called 'rapamycin', and this is the source of what may become effective anti-ageing medications and supplements, but be wary at the moment.

Some patients stick in your memory for a lifetime. I was a surgical resident in a large hospital in the west of London slap under the final flight path into Heathrow Airport. The noise could be deafening. Sadly, the hospital was also the final flight path for some patients. As an aside, I loved the job and it came close to making me want to become a surgeon but I was exhausted for almost all of its six months. It was a punishing roster where you could go days and nights on duty with no break. The residents' living quarters were situated between the Florence Nightingale-style wards, which were themselves connected by wide, high-ceilinged corridors. One incredibly busy night for emergencies had my registrar – an Australian who's now a successful surgeon in Melbourne – in one theatre, while I was in another taking out an inflamed appendix with appropriately anxious nurses and an anaesthetist looking on at the Scottish scalpel-wielding novice. At about 3 a.m. I got back to my room, undressed and collapsed into bed. What felt like moments later my pager went off with a crash alarm, indicating someone had gone into cardiac arrest, so I had to run. I dashed out of the room thinking it was just after 3 a.m., pulling on my scrubs as I catapulted into the corridor – to discover I'd slept in to 8.30 a.m. and the corridor was in rush hour. I've had nightmares of being netherly exposed in public places ever since.

Anyway, where was I? Oh yes, another memory seared in my brain from that time. I was called to see a man on the ward. He was a patient of the other 'firm' or surgical team who we covered when they were off duty. The man was around 40 years old and a couple of days post op – these were the times before hospital managers were obsessed with bed-days and getting people out as fast as possible. The curtains were drawn (no privacy – this was a ward with maybe 30 beds in two lines). The man looked as if he was smiling. He wasn't. He was terrified and the smile was the result of the muscles in his face being in spasm. His jaw was locked tight. I'd never seen tetanus before, only read about it in textbooks. In an appalling failure of surgical safety, he had somehow become infected with a soil organism called *Clostridium tetani* which, when it grows in your body, produces a toxin causing muscles to contract relentlessly. This man, whose name I can't remember, died despite all we tried to do for him.

In 1964, tetanus was one of the reasons for an expedition by Canadian researchers to Easter Island – or Rapa Nui, which is also the name of the Polynesian people who've been on the island for 800 years. This expedition was to transform the study of ageing and the later discovery of medications which might halt the ageing process and perhaps even rejuvenate us. The Canadians had to go by ship since it was to be another three years before this island, which is more than 2000 kilometres away from any other inhabited island, was to have an airport. The remoteness of this place, its isolated population and of course Rapa Nui's massive stone statues fascinated the Canadian scientists. On board was a specialist in infections and bugs – Montreal microbiologist Dr Georges Nógrady. One of the things he found odd was that unimmunised Rapa Nui went around barefoot yet didn't seem to come down with tetanus. He suspected there might be something in Easter Island's soil that fought germs. He was right. According to legend, despite taking samples from around the island, Nógrady couldn't find much in the way of *Clostridium tetani* which he would have if he'd looked at backyards in Quebec. When Dr Nógrady got back, he gave soil samples to a pharmaceutical company which is now part of Pfizer. They found the soil contained a bacterium called *Streptomyces hygroscopicus,* which manufactured a compound that fought against fungi like *Candida albicans* which causes 'yeast' infections. They named the substance after Rapa Nui: rapamycin. These days it's also called sirolimus.

But rapamycin was much more. It has anti-cancer effects and suppresses the immune system to the extent that today sirolimus and its pharmaceutical offspring are used to help kidney transplant recipients avoid rejection and may be useful in the therapy of some malignant tumours. It has side effects, though, such as increasing the risk of infection and poor blood sugar control, leading to type 2 or adult onset diabetes in some people.

So it might seem odd that rapamycin in some research circles has been heralded as the first compound to increase lifespan and maybe even healthy lifespan at that.

The next few paragraphs are a bit technical but give you a deeper understanding of how and why we age and the challenge of finding a drug that will slow down ageing and perhaps even reverse it. They explain why lifestyle can speed or slow ageing and help you decide whether someone's trying to sell you snake oil promising everlasting youth.

Scientists quickly became fascinated and searched for and found the molecular target of rapamycin in the body – calling it, unromantically, TOR (Target Of Rapamycin). In mammals it's called mTOR (mammalian Target Of Rapamycin). Since then, TOR has taken on far greater significance than just being the target of an Easter Island soil compound. TOR turned out to be one of the most fundamental ways our bodies control metabolism, immunity and ageing at a cellular level and is probably an ancient biochemical pathway. It's in organisms from yeast to humans.

TOR at its core is a complex set of switches which turn metabolism up and down, the multiplication and growth of cells on and off – including in muscles and the immune system – and, indirectly, drives ageing. One reason for the effect on ageing is that when mTOR is switched on, our cells go into overdrive and when they do, the energy factories in our cells – the mitochondria – spew out pollution. However, instead of smoke, their crap is free radicals – the unstable molecules which cause biological rusting (oxidative stress) and therefore ageing. The mTOR pathway is a highly sensitive nutrient sensor tuned to the carbs and protein we're eating. When we fast, mTOR is switched down like the volume control on your phone. When we gorge ourselves, it's switched on and amped up, increasing the sugar, fat and protein in the blood, ready for our body to grow either visibly or at a molecular level.

There's another reason mTOR can accelerate, slow or even reverse ageing.

Putting out the garbage

#notjustonsundaynights

You don't have to be old for bits of your body to wear out, but if the worn-out parts aren't replaced or fixed then you might become old sooner than you'd planned. Long before you see the visible manifestations of getting old, there's a process of wearing out and renewal inside our cells, especially the mitochondria – the energy factories and messaging centres. When our mitochondria clap out, so does the upkeep of the cells they're fuelling and just as the plastic garbage bags build up on the pavement when the bin-men are on strike, so does garbage inside our cells. The amazing thing about this mTOR pathway is that it senses when it's time to put out the bins, especially when we're young. Well, in fact, the process isn't really like putting out the garbage. When the body recognises that its useful stuff has become garbage, it starts to act like a molecular Marie Kondo. This kind of Kondo decluttering is called 'autophagy' and Marie would love it, if she could pull her head out of strangers' cupboards long enough. It's a process of gobbling up, recycling and renewing.

Sounds great, but just like Marie Kondo when she's on fire demanding to know whether we really love some piece of crap, so mTOR can get distracted and not attend to the molecular mess. Our behaviour and lifestyle are often what distracts it. When mTOR is fired up, there's no time or energy to be spared for autophagy because the focus is on growth and as a result the garbage builds up. Which is fine if it's just for a wee while but if it goes on and on like it does in an adolescent male's bedroom, it can be bad news.

I need to pause for a moment, because in the search for simple solutions to a complex process like ageing, there's one biological truth that at best can be disappointing and at worst dangerous to forget.

The words and phrases to describe this are: balance, harmony, push and pull, and the technical one, homeostasis. It's rare for any process in our bodies to be a one-way street.

If we produce more sugar (glucose) in our blood during our morning jog, there's a balancing process to take glucose out of our blood after breakfast and pack it away for next time. Same with fats and protein. Same with stimulating and settling down our immune system or the activity of the nerve networks in our brains. Remember this, because we need to be careful about what we wish for.

When you stop or inhibit mTOR from firing up, the garbage gets recycled (autophagy switches on), protein, glucose and fat metabolism start to go in a healthy direction, and in many animals and certainly yeast, lifespan and probably healthy lifespan goes up.

Sounds great but there's always the balance thing to take into account.

What holds back mTOR from firing up? Fasting, rapamycin and a growing list of other substances often called 'rapalogs'. But before I get to them, let's look at what gets mTOR going, since it starts to explain why how and what we eat helps us live younger for longer.

Why stuffing our faces stuffs up staying young

#anotherhelping
#inhalingleftovers
#welljustalittlethanks

A wee nibble: Eating too much fires up your body to go into a building phase, including depositing fat in all too visible places, encouraging cells to multiply and accelerating ageing.

You don't need to hear me going on yet again about my lousy self-control when it comes to food, but chronically overeating has scary side effects deep inside our cells.

Explanations like these are a bit like the warning for tourists – you can see all of Rome in a day, some of it in a week and none of it in a lifetime. It won't take me long to explain what's going on but underneath is mind-boggling complexity, which I'll leave until later because that's what mugs us when we buy into simple solutions.

As I've said before, mTOR is a nutrient-sensing machine. When food comes in, mTOR finds out and throws the switch on, packing these nutrients away through protein manufacture, sugar (glucose) storage, and provoking cells to multiply and get bigger. While it's doing this, there's no time or energy for cleaning up the mess. That's a between-meal thing. This is homeostasis at work in a healthily eating individual.

However, when you or I chronically overeat, mTOR goes into overdrive. Fat cells expand. Fat gets deposited in the liver. Insulin, which drives glucose out of the blood into cells, doesn't work as well (insulin resistance) and growth factors are turned on, as is unhelpful overactivity of the immune system (inflammation which can irritate arteries, cause atherosclerosis, speed tissue damage and degenerate the brain). The result? Well, you knew this already but now you know why there are higher risks of diabetes, heart disease, dementia and cancer. Overeating can disrupt homeostasis – the healthy push and pull of the mTOR system – and the result is more diseases of ageing and indeed ageing itself.

This push and pull is partly controlled by two switches, mTORC1 and mTORC2, and the one which has obsessed scientists is mTORC1 because it drives this overdrive and growth mode. The flip side is that if you could wrestle mTORC1 to the ground, you might stay younger longer.

That's where rapamycin comes in.

Rapamycin and staying young

#itdepends

Rapamycin – this natural substance from Easter Island – is a very odd medication. First thought to be an anti-fungal drug for treating infections like candida, it also suppresses the immune system and under its pharmaceutical name – sirolimus – has helped to save countless people with kidney transplants from organ rejection. Drugs developed from rapamycin like everolimus also show promise as anti-cancer treatments.

It does your head in, though, when you hear that this potentially toxic drug increases lifespan in animal experiments. WTF?

Rapamycin is like a wet blanket for mTORC1. In science-speak, it inhibits mTORC1. When an animal or cells in a dish are given rapamycin, the body works less hard at producing fats and protein and switches to clean-up mode – autophagy – allowing for a spot of rejuvenation and renewal. In fact, this may include the brain, where autophagy is important for cognitive function. Mind you, rapamycin doesn't easily pass from the blood to the brain. Dementia and Parkinson's disease may in part be the result of failed autophagy.

If you take rapamycin long term in high doses, it increases the risk of high blood sugars and diabetes, not to mention nasty infections from the immune suppression. That's thought to be because it isn't a 'clean' mTORC1 inhibitor. Used for long enough, it also inhibits mTORC2, which is the yang to mTORC1's yin. The proponents of using rapamycin to slow ageing say that low doses work better and that perhaps it should be taken intermittently rather than every day. The reasoning is that repeated, small nudges might keep ageing homeostasis off-balance. A successful anti-ageing strategy is likely to be one that restores our bodies to a youthful homeostasis. If you constantly drive ageing pathways down a one-way street, the body will resist because it's affecting countervailing processes which, while they might speed ageing, are also essential for health. For example, while accumulating garbage in the brain is doubtless bad for it, you also need the growth switch of mTOR for healthy nerve function and networks.

Rapamycin is too blunt a tool and more rapamycin is certainly not better. Hence some new biotech companies and their investment bankers believe that a cocktail may hold promise.

The Negroni approach

#cocktailsforever

Rapamycin turns off one of the master switches for ageing. While that might seem to be a good thing, it's a bit like turning out the light in your kitchen by going to the fuse box and cutting off the power to the whole house. It disrupts all kinds of other things. It's certainly true with mTOR, because it does so much more than control how quickly we fall apart. That's why researchers and biomedical entrepreneurs have developed rapamycin-like drugs – rapalogs – which work distantly from the master switches, further into the chemical wiring that's more focused on ageing mechanisms. In other words, if you want to turn off the kitchen light, hit the light switch in the kitchen itself.

You see, being so central to the way our body works, mTOR, like some old fart in a gentlemen's club, is resistant to change, so you have to bypass the resistance and it could be that gentle prods from different sides could work better.

For example, one placebo-controlled trial gave reasonably healthy people aged over 65 a short, six-week course of two rapalogs together versus dummy medications, and found that people on the active cocktail had better functioning immune systems. The participants' anti-viral genes were switched on, they had fewer infections in the following 12 months and, when given a flu shot, had an enhanced response. The main side effect was diarrhoea and they seemed to avoid the toxic mTORC2 imbalance I just mentioned.

There's a growing list of cocktail ingredients which might work better together than by themselves because they trigger different ageing genes rather than targeting one specific process, which by itself might provoke the body to oppose in its natural search for balance and homeostasis. Low dose rapamycin with metformin may be promising, as might adding rifampicin. Rifampicin's day job is as an antibiotic but it may also prolong lifespan. Another hopeful is allantoin, a natural substance in our bodies which is produced during exercise, helps wound healing, and is used as a drug in creams to soothe skin rashes.

There is also a list of drugs normally used for other purposes but which may increase autophagy, for example: valproic acid (epilepsy and migraine), lithium (bipolar disorder), trehalose (a food ingredient), spermidine (found in lots of plant-based foods), urolithin A (produced by a healthy gut microbiome and increased by berries, some nuts and pomegranate juice), and then of course there's rapamycin.

However, two of the leading non-drug candidates are very natural indeed: dietary restriction and the Mediterranean diet. A few of these substances are released by a traditional Mediterranean or plant-based diet and it's clear that dietary restriction plays in the same sandpit as rapamycin.

More pills to sell you – NAD+ precursors

#notcrackedityet

Quick take: I'll explain more below but taking supplements which boost NAD+ in your cells makes a lot of biological sense and seems to work in mice. But for some reason human studies have only shown minor benefits if any. No harm apart from skin flushing but negligible benefit. So if you're thinking of spending your money on a bottle of NR or NMN (don't buy online, by the way) then read on. One day they might find a way.

Why did I say don't buy online? You just don't know what you're getting. Studies of online pharmaceuticals have shown a very high level of fraud and contamination. At least in your local pharmacy you're more likely to be able to look at the bottle and reassure yourself that the regulator, the Therapeutic Goods Administration (TGA), has at least received the manufacturer's data on the product. But even then there are few guarantees since the TGA rarely checks that what the company says is in the bottle, actually is.

The theory behind NAD+ precursor supplementation: A precursor is the raw material from which a substance is made in your body. NAD+ is really important in our cells. It's basically a helper molecule that assists energy regulation and production, protection against free radicals (oxidative stress), communication inside cells and between them, and mitochondrial health. In organs like the heart and kidneys which consume large amounts of oxygen, NAD+ is thought to be even more important. Your kidneys in particular are pretty good clocks of biological age. So a lot of roads point to NAD+ and many researchers believe it's central to ageing – or at least should be. In some respects it, like other potential anti-ageing substances, mimics the effects of dietary (calorie) restriction particularly in the way it's involved with homeostasis – the balance thing – in mitochondria.

Various stresses and imbalances in the body are associated with reduced levels of NAD+ including being older and coronary heart disease. There is evidence that as you age NAD+ becomes less available to your cells. You've got to be a bit wary, though, of assuming that because something declines with ageing that it's causing ageing. A good example is testosterone (see Does Testosterone Have Balls when It Comes to Ageing?). While testosterone levels do fall with age, it's probably a sign of other things going on rather than being at the core of ageing.

So replacing testosterone, or its precursor DHEA, has been disappointing in terms of reversing the effects of ageing in otherwise healthy men.

NAD+, however, is much closer to ageing headquarters than testosterone.

There are two ways the body makes NAD+. One is a self-contained manufacturing process using the body's own supplies of a protein building block (amino acid) called tryptophan. The other is using vitamin B3 absorbed (or as the scientists like to say, 'salvaged') from your diet. The evidence is that this so-called salvage route is the most important for keeping NAD+ high in organs which need it, like muscles, heart and kidneys. This interest in precursor supplements brings us to vitamin B3. Also known as niacin, B3 is a mixture rather than a single substance, and one in the mix is nicotinamide riboside (NR), which is the commonest supplement (precursor) used to raise NAD+ levels. Another NAD+ precursor supplement is nicotinamide mononucleotide (NMN). Giving precursors as supplements aims to disrupt a person's homeostasis – metabolic balance – back towards youth by forcing the manufacture of NAD+. In fact, in lab animals and in human studies, that's exactly what NAD+ precursors do. NAD+ levels – or at least the signs of NAD+ metabolism – do rise significantly. Sounds great and it is the first step. The next stage, though, is finding out whether artificially boosting NAD+ levels makes any difference.

Those mice again: In lab animals, raising NAD+ levels has shown benefits such as improved cardiovascular function, rejuvenated mitochondrial activity, increased aerobic capacity, improved insulin sensitivity (ability to pull glucose out of the blood), less body fat and more muscle.

Those damned humans again: Placebo-controlled trials of NAD boosters in humans often suffer from being too small and badly designed to find the answers, but when you look at the trials as a whole in healthy adults of various ages and various BMIs, the results so far point in the same direction. The good news is that the precursors don't have many side effects apart from some skin flushing and appear safe. The bad news is that the benefits are hard to see. One study suggested a trend to improved cardiovascular health, such as more flexible arteries and reduced blood pressure, but these benefits were not statistically significant. Another study suggested increased fat-free body mass, especially in women, but oddly no accompanying increase in muscle mass which is what you'd expect. In general, mitochondrial function isn't improved after precursor supplementation, nor is muscle loss (even though muscle metabolism seems to go up). In most studies, body composition is unchanged, as are blood fats, kidney function, insulin sensitivity or levels of inflammation.

Disappointing but it's maybe too early to trash the idea because it's a mystery why animal research isn't translating into humans. It may be that larger, better designed trials are needed with more potent supplements. Or it may be that NAD+ is either the wrong target or again, like the other anti-ageing hopefuls, the human body finds ways to go back to what seems like an unhealthy homeostasis. If this is the case, it could be that precursors should be tested in combination with other compounds or lifestyles such as intense exercise, a diet high in bioactives and calorie reduction. The other strategy that could pay off, as mentioned before, is intermittent therapy to keep our bodies guessing.

Cocktails, the Mediterranean diet and frugality may go together

#allroads

A morsel: Dietary restriction works in a similar way to rapamycin. It slows down metabolism, reduces physical stress on cells and therefore slows or reverses ageing inside bodies and may even allow rejuvenation. It's not a magical route to always-on youth, just as resveratrol, metformin and rapamycin aren't. However, some think it could be an important addition to the cocktail along with – when you do eat – the Mediterranean dietary pattern, which is the mother of all cocktails.

Greek Australians – possibly the second-longest-lived people in the world – who are devout members of the Orthodox Church have around 100 frugal or fast days a year. Some writers have made a fortune out of telling us to fast on a regular basis. Humans have ancient genetic programs designed for intermittent fasting when we were hunter-gatherers but, having said that, life expectancy in the Stone Age was thought to be around 28, so be careful what you wish for. I'm a little cute in that observation because common causes of death would have been injury, violence and parasitic infections such as malaria and schistosomiasis. Even so, there is something to dietary restriction and when you look at what it does to our biochemical pathways – surprise surprise – restricting calories, like rapamycin, inhibits mTORC1 and switches cells to conservation mode, reducing their propensity to grow and multiply, lowering metabolic (oxidative) stress in our mitochondria, and allowing the garbage to be recycled (autophagy).

Dietary restriction has its practical limits but is a part of the mix.

Which brings us back to the Mediterranean dietary pattern. Let me refresh your memory if you read my previous book, *So You Think You Know What's Good For You?*, and if you haven't yet, here are some of the key takeaways.

It's called a dietary pattern because it's more than the individual foods. It's the way you cook, the ingredients used and how you eat. And when you look at what's cooked up, a fair proportion of the micronutrients in the Mediterranean dietary pattern are being recognised as having anti-ageing effects. Some researchers fresh from the lab are touting drug combinations – even perhaps intermittently – as the best approach to anti-ageing, but that's actually what happens each time you eat a diet high in plant-based foods, especially the colourful and red ones cooked in extra virgin olive oil.

There probably isn't a one-size-fits-all Mediterranean diet as such, since there are so many different nations and cultures on the Mediterranean shoreline. What people usually refer to as 'the Med diet' is how traditional Cretans eat or ate: lashings of extra virgin olive oil, which has a high concentration of bioactive anti-ageing compounds, not much red meat, a lot of vegetables and leafy plants, garlic and onions, fennel and fresh herbs and spices.

When you use extra virgin olive oil in cooking – especially with red vegetables – you release powerful compounds like polyphenols which include flavonoids and others which are increasingly recognised as counter-balancing the ageing pathway. Olive oil helps our bodies absorb and use some of these compounds, probably assisted by vinegar, which has beneficial effects on the microbiome by encouraging bacteria that produce healthy fatty acids. Fresh herbs like oregano, cumin and coriander assist too, along with onions, garlic, parsley and even capers. Some Asian cuisines have similar chemistry.

Research has also shown that the levels of polyphenols are raised by chopping vegetables like tomatoes and capsicum and adding olive oil and vinegar. Grilling gently in olive oil also works, an effect which isn't seen with sunflower oil, for example. The idea here is using complexity and variety in natural ingredients.

Garlic, onions, leeks, chives and shallots are all part of the allium family, the consumption of which is associated with reduced risks of various cancers. Stir-frying garlic may be best for retaining its active compounds, which is handy since pre-cooking garlic and onions in olive oil before adding the other ingredients is common in Mediterranean recipes. Adding tomatoes and sometimes chopped carrots to that mix – sofrito – really does amp up bioactives such as beta carotene and lycopene, flavonoids and biophenols which tend to depend on each other for optimal effects. Low levels of lycopene and other carotenoids are associated with lower cognitive function and premature death from all causes. The microbiome is also important. For instance, it produces butyrate, which helps to push a biochemical pathway called Nfr2/ARE which reduces oxidative stress and inflammation, slows tissue ageing, protects the brain and helps with a healthy level of cell death (apoptosis).

Studies of large groups of people have shown that populations who adhere closely to the Mediterranean dietary pattern have lower rates of mild cognitive impairment and dementia, and if there ever was a disease of ageing, it's dementia. A study of 23 developed nations showed that the higher the level of combined flavonoid intake in their diets, the lower the prevalence of dementia. This was controlled for income, education and other factors. Vitamin intake had no effect. Another study, following more than 1300 people aged over 65 for five years, found the group with the highest intake of flavonoids had half the risk of dementia and that was controlled for gender, education level, weight and vitamin C intake.

So if you think you can get round all this by chucking supplements down your throat before breakfast, think again. There is no bottle of pills in any pharmacy that comes close and pretty much no evidence that antioxidant supplements in pharmaceutical doses have any benefits at all for anyone apart from the manufacturer or the pharmacy owner. The secret is in the immense complexity of food, in ingredients like herbs and the dishes we cook.

Then there's how you cook. The Cretan and Greek way is do it slowly.

It's best to avoid high temperature cooking, which causes a lot of browning and caramelisation – barbecues, high temp grilling, etc. The reason is that high temperatures can produce pro-ageing compounds called advanced glycation end products (AGEs). The low-AGE recipe includes slow cooking with moisture (after marinating in vinegar or lemon juice – an acidic mixture), with lots of vegetables which are naturally low in AGEs even when grilled. For instance, roasted or grilled chicken has around four times the level of AGEs compared to poached or steamed chicken. AGEs can also accumulate in your body and no-one is too sure what effect that has on staying young.

Then there's intermittent Greek frugality which, in theory, should also inhibit the mTOR pathway. There is a lot of interest in intermittent interventions whether it's dietary restriction or anti-ageing drugs because tapping the pedal now and again may give the best chance to restore you to a youthful homeostasis. To change my metaphor, think of the body as a stubborn adolescent who refuses to do stuff when they're being ordered to do so or constantly nagged. They have to be cajoled and encouraged, and exasperated parents of teenagers learn to choose their battles. You don't want the mTOR pathway to lock in resistance to change. Greek Orthodox fasts, especially on the islands, occur on as many as 100 days of the year where for a day they don't eat meat, fish or dairy, just plant-based foods, often grown in their backyards. It probably dates back to when we were hunter-gatherers and fasting was better known as going hungry. When there weren't any animals to eat, foraged plants would have been all they had to be going on with – vegan days by necessity not by choice. It's likely ancient religions didn't want followers to forget the hard times and not appreciate the good ones. There are different versions of frugality, such as Lent, Ramadan and Yom Kippur, but they don't have the relatively even spread through the year of the Greek Orthodox church. An agnostic approach could be to deny yourself meat, fish and dairy every Monday and Thursday. Vegans may read this and wonder if they have a problem with homeostasis because they're eating that way all the time. There is research into vegetarians at least, which is reassuring. A diet that's rich in plants is associated with a longer healthy lifespan.

But still, researchers, start-ups and investors want to find a pill that will combat ageing faster, better and more profitably (for them).

Substances that may save you from eating your veggies (not)

#maybe
#strawberryfieldsforever

Short one: Some researchers believe that for a single anti-ageing compound to work, it has to have a cocktail of actions on the body all on its own. In other words, it keeps the body from resisting an attack from a single direction by coming at ageing from different approaches. One such compound could be fisetin. Another may be quercetin.

Fisetin is a flavonol – a polyphenol – found in plant foods, particularly strawberries and apples. Sadly, it isn't well absorbed by itself but when studied in the test tube and lab animals (sounding familiar?), fisetin suppresses tissue-ageing inflammation and controls the pro-ageing pro-oxidants – advanced glycation end products (AGEs) – produced in high temperature cooking that I've talked about before. Fisetin also inhibits cell death caused by oxidative stress (oxycytosis), may increase a neurotransmitter in the brain called acetylcholine (reduced in Alzheimer's disease), might encourage nerve growth, be good for the microbiome, and be a senolytic (see You Don't Want Bad Neighbours). One researcher – possibly missing the irony – has even described fisetin as able to mimic the effects of whole, plant-based foods.

#FFS

Fisetin-fed mice show improved memory, increased lifespan and reduced levels of age-related brain pathology. In mouse models of Parkinson's disease, fisetin increases dopamine levels in the brain, which is what Parkinson's medications do. In monkeys, combining fisetin with an anti-leukaemia drug, dasatinib, cleared old cells. And if all that isn't enough, fisetin seems to protect the heart from damage and reduces the toxicity of high glucose (sugar) levels in the blood. Some cancer researchers think fisetin could protect against the side effects of chemotherapy, but some oncologists believe that both fisetin and quercetin could actually lower the effectiveness of chemo by providing too much protection against damage.

Trouble is that there have been very few good studies in humans, fisetin doesn't dissolve easily in water and isn't absorbed well, and there's no patent so drug companies haven't invested in studies of it, although some groups are working on ways to make fisetin more bioavailable.

Quercetin is a plant pigment and a flavonol particularly found in red onions and their peel. One study suggests that organic red onions have more quercetin due to organic farmers' soil management practices. Like fisetin, quercetin has all kinds of effects in the lab but, while more bioavailable, is thought to be weaker than fisetin. In human studies so far, it's only convincing effect is to lower blood pressure although on the downside, it could interfere with blood thinners such as warfarin and aspirin.

But let's get to another source of ageing – useless but toxic old cells – and fisetin may be handy to help get rid of them.

You don't want bad neighbours

#grumpyoldbastards
#cellularfarting
#hitandrun

Quick take: Another cause of ageing throughout the body is that some clapped out cells refuse to die. What they do is hang around in the 'hood like a bored, grumpy neighbour who just sits there doing nothing but complaining and ringing up the cops when there's a party on. The cellular equivalent is that these grumpy, useless cells do molecular wet farts that damage the healthy cells around them, making them age. They're called senescent cells and a hot area of research is finding ways to get rid of them – senolytics. At the time of writing, though, these drugs and drug cocktails are not ready for showtime despite what some anti-ageing entrepreneurs might tell or sell you. One reason is complexity. There are lots of different senescent cells doing different kinds of wet farts, so finding a single treatment is a tough ask. A second reason is that a healthy body needs some senescent cells, which means you may not want to get rid of them all. It's that balance-homeostasis thing again but here's a guide to what's going on and what you can do while you wait.

I first came across the concept of senescent cells when I met Professor Jan van Deursen, a Dutch-American biologist who was then at the world-renowned Mayo Clinic in Rochester, Minnesota. It was late January, when Rochester is so cold that you walk between the Mayo's buildings via underground corridors. People from around the world flock to the clinic for its world-leading care, as do researchers for its science, and medicine is pretty much all there is to do in this town. The hospital is surrounded by hotels where, to save resources, preparation for medical procedures can take place. The apocryphal story is getting a knock on the door and thinking it's room service, when what confronts you is a nurse sent there by a practical joker to give you an enema. As usual, I digress.

Van Deursen was one of the pioneers of senescent cell research and some of the metaphors I use are his (the wet farts are mine).

Stress causes cells to lose their mojo. It's the oxidative stress or biological rusting I've often mentioned, which is part of living and made worse by a lousy diet and lifestyle. It's also the social and economic stress of deprivation, which shortens telomeres – the protective ends of our chromosomes and molecular biological clocks – the longer your telomeres, the better. It can even be physical stress from injury, wounds or radiation. Cancer genes (oncogenes) can trigger senescence as can DNA damage and mitochondrial dysfunction. Senescence can be the result of attack from an inflamed immune system, perhaps provoked by environmental issues such as air pollution.

However, sometimes cells are programmed to stop working and it's a healthy response. For example, you find senescent cells in wounds, which are a sign the body is trying to control the healing process so you don't get overgrowth of scar tissue. You find senescent cells in embryos because the embryo or foetus is sculpting arms and legs and needs to stop growth in every direction. You find senescent cells in malignant tumours. Sometimes they're part of the cause and sometimes they're an attempt to halt uncontrolled growth and spread.

Having said all that, senescent cells are heavily involved in ageing and could be targets to slow it down. The process, as far as it's understood at the moment, goes something like this. The stresses and strains of living, and the declining effectiveness of the immune system to vacuum up debris, cause the accumulation of cells that have simply stopped working and dividing as they used to. But they don't sit there quietly. They secrete substances that cause nearby healthy cells to age faster themselves. They also irritate the immune system but instead of irritating immune cells to clear out the senescent cells, the inflammation just makes the ageing effect worse. Some call this the chronic inflammatory state of ageing. Sometimes the cells' secretions can make it easier for cancer cells to grow and spread. The secretions can act like a repellent to immune cells sniffing around to devour them. The thing is that there isn't just one kind of senescent cell or one pattern of secretions. Even so, the two main targets of researchers trying to develop so-called senolytics are firstly the cells themselves and secondly their secretions, or wet farts if you like my scatological metaphor. Interestingly, there is some evidence that COVID-19 disease increases senescent cell secretions.

Here's some of the evidence supporting senescent cells as anti-ageing targets.

When mice that are genetically programmed for rapid ageing are given a senolytic designed to clean out senescent cells, the animals age more slowly. The converse is also true, suggesting cause and effect: namely, when senescent cells are transplanted into healthy tissue, it starts to show age-related degeneration. When you look at humans and measure the senescent cells in their bodies, the burden correlates with age-related diseases in the heart, lungs, brain, liver and hormone systems.

There's a growing list of potential senolytics from animal and test-tube studies. For example, the combination of the anti-leukaemia drug dasatinib with quercetin cleans out senescent cells. Anti-lymphoma drugs called BCL-2 inhibitors – and in particular a new one called navitoclax – do this too as, potentially, can a cell therapy called CAR-T where immune cells are taught to attack receptors (lock and key mechanisms) on the surface of senescent cells. In the same way, some think special vaccines could work, perhaps aiming at senescent cells in fat tissue. Metformin might be a senolytic, as might fisetin. At the time of writing, there's quite a long list of human clinical trials into senolytics.

Hit and run: As you can imagine, throwing anti-cancer drugs at ageing might have mixed results with toxic side effects ('off-target effects') on the immune system. That's why some researchers claim that a hit and run approach to dosing might work with, say, a once a fortnight treatment. The rationale is that it takes more than a week for senescent cells to accumulate, so you might only need the cleaner to come in every so often.

So what can you do in the meantime?

Well, reduce oxidative stress by what you eat and how you cook it. Eat plants. Don't smoke them. Try to inhale clean air. Lower the amount of fat on your body to reduce the level of immune activation. If you have an autoimmune condition like rheumatoid arthritis which speeds ageing through inflammation, make sure you're on medications to modify the disease (steroids are not disease modifiers). Avoid too much sun because that's a cause of senescence too. And by all means eat foods high in fisetin and quercetin, but maybe hang on a bit before taking them as supplements until there's more evidence that taking them by themselves in high doses is safe and effective.

Which leaves exercise and having strong muscles.

PART 4

Outrunning the clock – staying young with exercise

#keepitsimple
#savehopeforhype

Short of time? You can buy up all sorts of garbage in pharmacies and online in the hope that it'll save you effort and time. But that's what it'll be: hope. It's not that senolytics, mTORC1 inhibitors and NAD+ precursors won't pay off one day, but while you hope that they will, you can't ignore what definitely does work to keep you young and ultimately living longer. Along with diet and how you cook and eat, exercise – physical activity – is very high on the list and, in fact, is a senolytic in its own right. In general more exercise is better, more intense is even better (and could save you time) but whatever you do must include muscle strengthening. People who exercise reduce their chances of premature death by up to 34 per cent. The fitter you are, the lower your risk of dying of cancer. Many of the benefits from exercise happen over the three or four days after you've taken it. Physical activity drops your blood pressure, your triglycerides and level of inflammation, and raises your good (HDL) cholesterol. All good news but it means it's better taking exercise every day or second day, rather than waiting till the weekend and suffering a 'benefits gap'. Exercise which builds muscle while you're younger makes you look better; it's a huge investment for the future if you keep it up. Strong muscles can prevent diabetes and the decline to frailty which all too often makes late life a misery leading to premature death. At age 50, moderate activity gets you two years extra and heavy activity four years, and also can deliver you several more years of healthy life. At age 80 there are still around two years extra to be had from a combination of aerobic and strengthening exercise. If you've participated in sports at a high level, you can gain up to six years of life and the diseases you'll eventually die of come on ten years later than people who haven't played sports to a high level, especially if your alcohol consumption is low.

Before I dive deep, it's probably time to step back and look at what I've talked about a few times, namely homeostasis. It's the balance of forces in our bodies and when everything's in harmony and in its place, we have health and wellbeing. When homeostasis is knocked off its ledge, all sorts of things happen. When balance is lost in our blood fats or control of blood pressure, we get heart disease. When balance is lost in blood sugar control and body fat, we get diabetes. And when balance is lost at the cellular level, we lose our youth and turn into biological degenerates. Some experts have argued that ageing is a disruption of homeostasis. So starting young is about shoring up the balance.

Stay with me on this because it helps to explain why exercise is so potent.

One group of researchers has argued that, at a cellular level, there are nine interrelated features of ageing all of which throw us off balance and stuff up homeostasis: our genome – our genes and DNA – becomes unstable; our telomeres lose control of their length and start to erode, leaving our chromosomes exposed; our genes alter their shape and structure and therefore their function (epigenetic changes); we don't monitor and respond to nutrients in our diet as well (nutrient-sensing – the mTOR pathway, in fact); we get imbalances in protein production (loss of proteostasis); our energy factories – the mitochondria – become dysfunctional; our cells become senescent; the stem cells which make new tissue clap out; and finally, cells don't talk to each other as well as they used to.

It's like the control room at the ill-fated Chernobyl nuclear power station (did you see the series, by the way?). One shitty thing after another happens because the underlying system falls apart and then it's a pathway to meltdown because these mechanisms of ageing are all about causing damage and responding badly to damage, and the net result is loss of homeostasis. To stay young, you've got to keep the underlying system in good shape and the forces of destruction counter-poised with the forces for good.

And exercise is great at that.

If you're not convinced and would still rather swallow your fisetin (which you could still do but on top of exercise), let me give you some of the evidence – which is pretty much entirely lacking so far for all the anti-ageing pills I've talked about, but is there in spades for exercise.

While I've been bagging animal research because it can fail to translate to humans, physical activity actually seems to work better in humans than in animals in the lab. Let's start with where we left the last section – senescent cells and senolytics. Regular physical activity, resistance training and moderate to high intensity cycling have all been shown to reduce the markers of senescent cells in people. In experimental rodents they've found lower levels of the wet farts (toxic secretions) as well. Resistance (strength) training may have the edge as a senolytic, but the evidence for life extension in good health is so strong for aerobic training as well, that mixing it up is the best strategy and that's reflected in most national exercise guidelines. The reasons exercise works at the cellular level include: reducing oxidative stress, increasing the clearance of garbage (autophagy), maintaining the length of the telomeres at the end of your chromosomes and therefore increasing genetic stability, and stopping cells from becoming senescent in the first place by killing them off as they're starting to age (programmed cell death or apoptosis).

A recent study at the Mayo Clinic confirmed this when they put older people through a structured exercise program two days per week for 12 weeks. They found reduced senescent cell biomarkers and lower levels of senescent cell secretory proteins.

A 21-year follow-up of runners aged 50 and older compared to non-runners found that 15 per cent of the runners had died compared to 34 per cent of the non-runners, and that allowed for the fact that people who exercise a lot generally don't smoke, drink much alcohol or have too much fat on their bodies.

Almost one in ten people who die before their time – globally – can blame physical inactivity for their premature mortality. A follow-up of 55,000 men and women found exercise was associated with a gain in healthy lifespan even if they were a smoker, overweight or drank a lot. The reduction in premature death from any cause in exercisers was between 30 and 45 per cent and added up to an extra three years of life on average, which increased to four years with more vigorous exercise.

If you look at the risk factors for living shorter older, lack of exercise is fourth after high blood pressure, smoking and raised blood sugar levels.

Which exercise?

There's a lot of discussion about which exercise is best and while there's a lot of evidence about runners because the intensity appears to be higher on average, the downside is that running isn't everyone's cup of tea and there can be issues with injury. Resistance training strengthens muscles as well as increasing aerobic capacity and both are important. Static cycling is good because it's probably a bit easier for high intensity interval training (HIIT).

So what's the aim? It seems clear from the scientific literature that the measure which correlates most closely with reductions in premature death and therefore living longer is cardiorespiratory fitness. Strong muscles count too. Cardiorespiratory fitness is associated with lower blood pressure, a healthier blood fat profile (higher HDL in particular), increased bone density, increased effectiveness of insulin at getting glucose out of your bloodstream (high glucose levels are toxic and pro-ageing), reduced risk of depression, improved thinking and memory and increased grey matter in your brain. Remind me which of the pills they're flogging to keep you young are proven to do all that in humans? Yep, none.

What's moderate and what's intense?

The scientific way of working this out is using the metabolic equivalent of task – the MET value of an exercise. It's the added burn of an exercise beyond sitting still; i.e. when your body's at rest (1 calorie per kilogram per hour). The number of METs which qualify for light, moderate or intense depends on your age and weight. On average a 6 MET exercise is moderate and an 8 MET is fairly vigorous. At age 80, again on average, moderate exercise is between 2 and 3 METs and vigorous is between 3 and 4. Brisk walking is around 4 METs, swimming's similar and jogging's about 8 METs. The aim is to burn at least 1000 calories per week exercising, ideally aiming for up to 3500 calories. So if you're 80 kg, then brisk walking burns about 320 calories an hour whereas jogging burns around 640 calories an hour. So if you can jog, it does take you further faster.

The time–intensity continuum

While the mortality benefits of exercise tend to kick in at 500 MET minutes per week, you should aim for over 900 MET minutes per week. To work out the METs you're earning, multiply the number of minutes you exercise by the MET value of that exercise. You can start to see why intensity is important because the higher the MET value of the exercise, the less time you spend getting through it. However, this can get unnecessarily complicated. Crudely and simply, if you're able to have a nice chat to your friend while out exercising, it ain't even moderate. Self-delusion is huge with exercise. In other words, you convince yourself that you're doing more than you actually are. Moderate is when you're sufficiently pushed that you're a bit out of breath and find conversation hard. If you're very unfit and overweight, that could be a walk to the shops. If you're fit and lean, you'll need more intense exercise to get to that level of breathlessness which also equates to your pulse and how close it is to maximum for your age. I'm not going to get into much more detail because you may have a medical condition that affects your safe exercise level. Being sensible is important and there are tables and charts if you want to be scientific about this. You can take your time to build up your fitness – taking advice from your physician in case there any risks you need to be aware of. The key is gradually and safely to increase your effort because if you can speed up your walking then you'll burn more in less time.

To give you another idea of the time–intensity continuum, a study of 400,000 Taiwanese men and women, followed for eight years using all-cause mortality as a measure, found that running for 5 minutes and 25 minutes were the health equivalent of walking for 15 minutes and 105 minutes.

A more recent randomised trial found that running was better than resistance training when it came to keeping those telomeres at the ends of your chromosomes at a youthful length. That doesn't mean that muscle training wasn't important, it's just that different forms of exercise fulfil different purposes.

Be progressive

Progressive in this sense isn't that you vote for the Greens. It's that you constantly increase the intensity of your exercise to match your improving aerobic fitness and muscle strength as measured, say, by your pulse rate and the weights you use or the number of sit-ups and push-ups in a certain time period. As you become fitter, it will take less time to burn the calories or in the same time you'll burn more.

HIIT vs MIT: HIIT is high intensity interval training and MIT is moderate intensity training. Most recommendations land on 45–60 minutes of MIT on most days of the week mixed with muscle-strengthening exercises. There are various protocols for HIIT but they generally involve 20 or 30 seconds of going flat out (sprints) followed by recovery time, repeated several times. Probably best done under supervision until you get it right and do it sensibly. The point is that HIIT and MIT both improve cardiorespiratory fitness to a similar extent. It's just that HIIT does it in less time each week.

The more the better, up to a point: There's lot of debate about whether there's a maximum amount of exercise beyond which you don't get additional benefits. Some believe that 50 MET hours a week is the upper limit, assuming you're not training for the Olympics. My advice is worry about the limit when you get there although a recent study from Denmark suggests that when it comes to *sports* exercise, 10 hours a week might be getting too much.

Never too late: Interestingly, the gain in years of life doesn't seem to be closely tied to the age at which you start exercising – there are extra years available regardless of age.

Do it daily: Here's why it needs to be daily rather than loading up your METs for the weekend. Think of exercise as a medication that only lasts in your body for a certain time. For example, you need to take antibiotics every six or eight hours because the body has eliminated a significant proportion of the earlier dose by then. With exercise, the benefits in terms of the cellular effects and, say, reductions in blood pressure may only last a day or two, at which point you need another dose to get you back on track, so to speak. Don't keep all your METs for the weekend.

Dietary restriction needs exercise: According to anti-ageing expert Professor Luigi Fontana, exercise is a really important component of dietary restriction for all the reasons above plus avoiding your background calorie burn dropping. It's another example of homeostasis at work where if you lower your calorie intake your body adjusts and lowers your metabolic rate to compensate. Exercise keeps up the calorie 'burn'.

What about your step count? The above gives you a better guide to exercise levels but if you're into step counting, the cut-off for avoiding premature death appears to be 7000 steps a day or more, from a recent US study at the time of writing.

But wait, there's more...

So you get the idea, exercise has more evidence to support living younger longer than any anti-ageing pill or supplement you can buy or be prescribed. But before we move on, here are more benefits to help keep you motivated and off the couch.

Cancer and exercise: Because of the cellular and hormonal effects of exercise, you're less likely to develop cancer – especially bowel and breast – if you exercise regularly; and if you do have cancer, treatment will be more effective and your quality of life improved.

Your brain and exercise: The more intense the exercise, the more it lifts your mood and improves your cognitive function. Another factor, though, is that often exercise studies are done with other people or in a gym where you might have to remember your reps and count a lot. So while you're creating healthy metabolic stress, which is good for neural connections and nerve growth, you also may be in a more cognitively stimulating environment.

School sport: Follow-up studies, particularly of women who were athletes at school, show enormous long-term gains in health and probably even larger effects on lifespan.

Get a grip

#notjustanarmwrestle

Strong muscles are essential for slowing down ageing and avoiding the slippery dip into frailty in your later years. Your muscles are also highly effective at metabolising blood sugar and keeping your insulin working well, which is why muscle strengthening can prevent diabetes.

There are multiple studies showing a relationship between the strength of your grip – hand grip strength – and a variety of conditions including dying prematurely. Before you rush off to increase your grip strength with specially designed springs or by hanging off monkey bars, it's not the strength of your forearm muscles that will make you live longer. Hand grip strength is really just a reflection of how much muscle you have on the upper and lower halves of your body. It's a simple, easy test to perform and gives an idea of how much work you need to do on your muscles in general. Just developing a steel-like handshake by itself won't cut it.

PART 5

Bugs, bowels and hormones

Anna Karenina and the microbiome

#keepyourbugsyoung
#keepawayfromvronskys

Quick one: The squillions of bugs in your bowel are almost certainly both passengers and drivers in the bus that's your body heading down the freeway away from youngness. Some researchers believe they can tell your age by looking at your microbiome. One day, they may find the actual bugs which could go into a 'stay young' probiotic pill but they're not there yet. However, there is stronger and stronger evidence of cause and effect from the microbiome when it comes to slowing ageing and things you can do right now which make a difference.

In researching this section, I came across microbiome researchers who talk about what they call 'the Anna Karenina Principle'. It comes from Leo Tolstoy's famous novel's opening lines:

'All happy families are alike; each unhappy family is unhappy in its own way.'

If you've read *Anna Karenina*, you'll know that there are actually no happy families in the book. However, that's not where the analogy goes when it comes to the microbiome because there are happy families in our bowels and happy (i.e. healthy) microbiomes are very similar to each other, whereas unhealthy patterns of bowel bugs are quite different depending on the person and their problems. A healthy microbiome helps to slow the ageing process, prevent the development of chronic diseases and possibly even the loss of muscle mass which leads to frailty near the end of the bus ride. Bottom line is good news. We know roughly what a healthy microbiome is composed of and how to create it. On the flip side, even though unhealthy, pro-ageing microbiomes vary a lot, we know what appears to cause them and at least in part how to make them healthier. And for once there's a growing body of real world research in humans rather than rats and mice.

To stay young as long as possible, our task is to keep the peace between the forces which push and pull us. That push and pull gives us the flexibility to adapt to our environment probably better than any other species on the planet. As time goes by, though, this balance – homeostasis – is steadily knocked out of kilter. As you've already found out, a lot of this book is about how that happens and how to restore a more youthful homeostatic profile. One result of disrupted homeostasis is that something called our innate immune system loses the plot, causing abnormal activation of certain immune cells, which in turn cause inflammation and tissue damage. Some call this 'inflamm-ageing'.

Our innate immune system is the body's first line of defence when there's a foreign invasion, say, of bacteria. Unlike the highly specific, targeted immunity that comes from a vaccine, the innate immune system is like World War 1 artillery fire creating a barrage of immune cells and secretions, supplied by increased blood flow, to kill the enemy before it gets too far. That's inflammation (with apologies to any immunologist reading this who'd prefer a wee bit more detail, but hey, I'm not sitting an exam, guys).

Nothing new away from the sun

While the current obsession with the microbiome is relatively recent, the idea that it may be central to ageing was put forward more than a century ago by the scientist who won a Nobel Prize in 1908 for his description of the innate immune system and the white blood cells involved – Elie Metchnikoff. Metchnikoff was Russian born but spent most of his career at the Pasteur Institute in Paris, studying micro-organisms and our response to them, including in the bowel. He hypothesised that ageing was the result of 'auto-intoxication' where the balance of friendly and unfriendly gut bacteria was lost, toxins were produced, and as a result the innate immune system was activated causing tissue damage and ageing. This was before molecular biology, before genomics and before all the investigative technologies that researchers have today. It was also before scientists understood the immense complexity and size of the gut's immune system, lined up like border guards along the lining (mucosa). Metchnikoff believed that lactobacilli were the answer to auto-intoxication by restoring a healthy balance and, in fact, he commercialised and promoted yoghurt as a potent source of these bacteria and as an anti-ageing product. Sadly, the yoghurt didn't work well on Metchnikoff, who slid into ageing and died in 1916 aged 71.

Our colonic clock

It looks as though you can tell the biological age of someone with reasonable accuracy by analysing their microbiome. We probably acquire our initial microbiome during pregnancy from the amniotic fluid and placenta and at birth from vaginal delivery. A baby's microbiome changes a lot in the first three years and is influenced by being breastfed versus formula, how many brothers and sisters you have, whether there are pets, exposure to fermented foods (Metchnikoff wasn't all wrong), and geography, travel, hospital stays and antibiotic prescriptions. After the age of around 20, the microbiome is fairly stable until it starts to deteriorate later in life or due to poor diet, disease and medication use.

Young and healthy people have forests of different kinds of organisms with huge diversity and fairly predictable families of bugs that do good things like produce substances called short chain fatty acids (SCFAs) which, among many functions, make the immune system more tolerant and less likely to fire up unnecessarily. They also reduce oxidative stress and probably influence the gut's incredibly complicated nervous system, which is thought to regulate how we absorb nutrients from the diet. These microbial families – or taxa – also shore up the lining of our gut, making it less leaky and therefore less likely to absorb toxins and pass them around the body. I said biological age because healthy older people can have the microbial signature of people a fraction of their age. Conversely, people who are becoming biologically old and frail have thinned-out forests with far less diversity. Their microbial families are biased towards damaging metabolism where irritating substances like bile acids, p-cresol and even ethanol and carbon dioxide build up.

Chicken or egg? Before I go on, what's not been fully sorted out yet is cause and effect. I said earlier that the microbiome could be both passenger and driver of the ageing bus. The bus may be badly driven, fuelled with dirty diesel, stuffing up the passengers. Equally the driver herself could be part of the microbiome guiding the bus to happier destinations and making it less polluting. All this means that sometimes you're heading for disappointment when trying to manipulate the microbiome. Our ignorance of how it all works in detail might end up with us inadvertently targeting the passengers rather than the drivers. May not be harmful, just frustrating.

Even so, probiotics should work against ageing, right?

Well, wrong, at least at the moment, partly because the anti-ageing effects come from taxa – massive groups of bacteria – of different kinds but which have similar metabolic profiles. Researchers are trying to see if there are, within these populations, specific bacteria which would do the job if given as a supplement but trials of such specific probiotic bacteria have not shown benefits – at least not yet. Interestingly, metformin (see Which Pill and Why?) works on the microbiome to increase SCFA production, which may be why it could have an anti-ageing effect. Over the next few years expect to see more and more microbiome-targeted therapies but in the meantime ...

A *prebiotic* approach does seem to work

The reason why people's microbiomes become less diverse and shift to a more pronounced state of inflamm-ageing is thought to be that people's diets become less diverse, containing more fat – especially saturated fats – and more refined carbohydrates. In fact, there are groups of bacteria in the bowel which are fairly tightly linked to chronic diseases like diabetes, cognitive impairment and frailty. This is even more exaggerated if someone is admitted to residential aged care with its often notoriously bad food. Antibiotics don't help either and can cause havoc in the microbiome. Low fat, high fibre diets, on the other hand, are associated with more diverse, healthier microbiomes. The prebiotic approach aims to maintain and increase the diversity of foods, with more fruit and vegetables, more protein from legumes and fish and less from red meat, more polyunsaturated and monounsaturated fats (olive oil) and less saturated fat. That pattern gives you a good dose of bioactives which interact with each other, enhancing their activity and profoundly influencing the microbiome.

A one-year study of more than 1000 older people across Europe gave them a diet like this – i.e. a Mediterranean diet – or put them in a control group who had their usual diet. A subset of 600 had their microbiome profile analysed. The controls decreased in biodiversity and the active group either maintained or increased theirs. The results showed increased production of short chain fatty acids in the Med diet people and lower production of damaging bile acid products, p-cresol and carbon dioxide. P-cresol is produced by bacteria in the bowel which help with protein breakdown and is raised in infections and kidney disease.

Those eating the intervention diet had lower markers of frailty, improved cognitive function, and lower levels of C reactive protein (CRP) – a marker of inflammation. This doesn't prove cause and effect but in the context of a randomised trial does give some confidence.

This doesn't just happen in the elderly. An eight-week randomised trial of the Mediterranean diet in 82 overweight or obese people who were otherwise healthy found evidence of increased short chain fatty acid production and lower levels of pro-inflammatory bacterial species.

Returning to Anna Karenina and an indication of where probiotic development might go, a large study of 2500 people, aged between 20 and 89 with a variety of diseases, conformed to the AK principle in that those with diseases like type 2 diabetes and inflammatory bowel disease had their own patterns of bowel bugs, whereas the healthy people had similar patterns of what the researchers presumed were protective organisms.

Anyway, you know what you need to do.

Does testosterone have balls
when it comes to ageing?

#takecaremachoman
#wannafeelyoungagain

Quick take: The role of testosterone is far from clear when it comes to staying young and living longer. Male animals, including humans, generally have shorter lives than females and there's a fair amount of evidence that living a life with testosterone on board is partly to blame. There's also evidence that drugs to prevent heart disease and diabetes reduce testosterone levels, and some wonder if that's an added benefit when it comes to saving lives. On the other hand, testosterone does decline with age and, in some studies, lower testosterone levels are associated with premature death. Long story short, unless you have a condition called hypogonadism where you're seriously short of testosterone and having symptoms, you need to be careful about testosterone or other anabolic steroid supplementation. They may not buy you extra lifespan.

My hashtags above may trivialise what are important issues for some men. Dr Matthew Dunn, a public health researcher at Deakin University, has been researching men's attitudes to ageing and the use of anabolic steroids. 'What we're hearing from men in their 40s and beyond is that they've delayed important milestones in their lives – things such as having kids – for career and social reasons and they feel their lives haven't been what they planned and want to restore a feeling of youth,' explains Dr Dunn. 'This becomes a driver to take steroids in the hope they'll look more muscular and masculine and feel younger. There's also frustration that they don't qualify for such medications on prescription and have to use the illegal market.'

Dr Dunn thinks there could be parallels with the revival of psychedelic drugs, which have become popular for people wanting to go through a life reset.

So, let me try to make sense of the science of using testosterone, since it's the natural anabolic steroid in both men and women.

Pretty much wherever you look in the animal kingdom, male animals live shorter lives than female ones. The easy assumption to make is that the one big difference between males and females is that males have more testosterone on board throughout life. Castration is a way of studying this because it removes most testosterone production. Castrated dogs and rats live longer than ones who are left with their testes. A fascinating study in Korea looked at the historical records of eunuchs who served as guards, servants and sometimes as trusted senior officials during the Chosun Dynasty from the 14th century. Small numbers, but what they found was that eunuchs lived significantly longer than non-castrated men, sometimes even into their 90s and 100s when the average lifespan was in the 50s or less. Yes, there could be other explanations such as lifestyle and income but it does fit with the non-human animal data.

Another study took data from 167,000 men and 194,000 women in what's called the UK Biobank, where they store lifestyle and medical information as well as gene sequencing on huge numbers of people. They looked for genes which control the production of testosterone and found that lifelong testosterone exposure to age 57 was indeed associated with reduced survival. This is testosterone from natural production within the body, not supplementation. The theoretical reasons that testosterone could be the cause of premature death are that its levels are linked to increased atherosclerosis and breast, prostate and uterine cancer. Testosterone may also be an immune suppressant. There is also evidence that medications which increase healthy lifespan, such as statins for lowering cholesterol, metformin for diabetes, and perhaps aspirin, are linked to lower testosterone levels, as might be a low animal fat diet.

On the other side of the ledger, there are many studies showing that the levels of testosterone and the raw material from which it's made, dehydroepiandrosterone (DHEA), decline with age and are associated with shorter lives. But most of the people with low levels are particularly unhealthy because of smoking, inactivity and poor diets. These studies are observational, meaning that there are limits to what you can infer about cause and effect from watching people, and most researchers in the field believe it's the unhealthy lifestyle that's the problem rather than the testosterone. Studies following large numbers of men have found that older men can have the testosterone levels of younger males and that's usually associated with good metabolic health and not being overweight or obese. One study of healthy ageing men found no age-related decline in testosterone at all. It was a smoking history, obesity and other medical conditions which were linked to lower testosterone levels.

In addition, it's not at all clear what the difference is between testosterone produced in the tissues of the body and testosterone absorbed from a patch in sometimes quite high doses.

This hasn't stopped the growth of a multibillion-dollar industry for testosterone or DHEA replacement therapy. Randomised trials in men have found no benefit in vitality, muscle strength or weight loss. There are small but short-lived improvements in sexual performance. Losing weight and getting some decent exercise will probably do more for you. There are small and mostly theoretical risks of heart disease and prostate cancer but most trials haven't gone on long enough to really know.

Adult onset hypogonadism is relatively rare and associated with symptoms including psychological changes, erectile dysfunction, loss of both libido and male pattern hair, breast enlargement and fragile bones. This is a situation where testosterone replacement does help.

In women? In healthy, young, physically active women, testosterone cream has been shown to improve aerobic running time and increase lean mass. Not a reason for young women to get into testosterone cream because safety is still an unknown. There is little evidence that testosterone in women increases the actual strength of muscles. That may be more of a role of female hormones.

In premenopausal women there is no link between a woman's levels of most hormones and sexual function including arousal. There may be a small association with testosterone levels but the researchers weren't sure it was a significant finding. Having said that, when researchers have brought together the available evidence, there is support for using testosterone patches to improve arousal and desire. But long-term safety hasn't been proven.

And what about oestrogen?

#itsironic

The take: The story with oestrogen and living younger longer has echoes of testosterone. First of all, the evidence is mixed and a bit confused (some experts might say the confusion is mine but I'll cop that). In theory, oestrogen should be good for ageing as it seems to reduce oxidative stress, but when you look at lifetime exposure to oestrogen produced in the body – what's called endogenous oestrogen – the more women are exposed to endogenous oestrogen, the higher their risk of heart disease, stroke and breast cancer. There are various ways to measure this. One is the number of menstrual periods a woman has, because each cycle produces a surge of oestrogen above background. So, for example, if a woman starts her periods later in adolescence, the rate of breast cancer reduces, as it does when she has children, especially if she breastfeeds and delays periods even further. Another way of measuring this is called reproductive lifespan, which is the number of years between periods starting (menarche) and finishing (menopause). By the way, these increased risks may have nothing whatsoever to do with oestrogen and be the fault of its companion hormone, progesterone, which also surges during menstruation. Then there's the question of taking oestrogen-only supplements (exogenous oestrogen) usually in the form of hormone replacement therapy (HRT) during and after the menopause. This is only advised for women who've had their womb removed (hysterectomy) because oestrogen unopposed by progesterone increases the risk of uterine cancer. Oestrogen-only HRT is good at reducing menopausal symptoms and maybe strengthening bones a little, without raising the risk of breast cancer or heart disease, but there's no evidence there's a longevity benefit.

There is, though, in the scientific literature a cruel irony for women; well, for female mice at least. A version of oestrogen called 17 α (alpha) oestradiol appears to make *male* mice live longer, especially when given in midlife. This doesn't occur in female or castrated mice and is unlikely to be the result of rodent males getting in touch with their female side. It's biology which has yet to be fully explained.

Women do it differently

#ageingthatis

Not quite Venus and Mars: Animals, especially humans, need to be complicated. If the way our internal machinery worked was simple, we'd be much more vulnerable to attack from toxic substances and infections than we are. So it's no surprise really that females seem to age differently from males and respond differently to lifespan-extending interventions, although as usual, what we know mostly comes from animal research. For example, across an astounding 36 species, dietary restriction appears to have greater benefits for females than males. One reason may be that it works better at protecting against age-related intestinal problems. I already mentioned 17 α oestradiol as only working on male mice with their testes still in place. Other possible life extenders such as rapamycin work better in female mice, while acarbose, aspirin and nordihydroguaiaretic acid (NDGA) appear to work a bit better in male mice. I haven't mentioned acarbose and NDGA before. NDGA extends lifespan in mice probably because it helps clear out the ageing garbage (see Putting Out the Garbage), and acarbose is a medication used to treat diabetes and reduces spikes in blood sugar. Males across various species may have less effective sugar (glucose) metabolism and high blood sugars are toxic and accelerate ageing. Which may explain acarbose's stronger effect. Another reason males and females age differently could be in our chromosomes. The lack of a second X chromosome in males may make us more susceptible to mutations. In other words, women have more back-up with the second X.

Antibiotics – living longer, living shorter

#itdepends

In a capsule: No-one will know for sure by how much, but the introduction of antibiotics in the 20th century significantly contributed to us living longer, maybe by several years, due to the cure of previously fatal pneumonia and other bacterial infections. With the misuse of antibiotics by doctors and farmers causing drug resistance, we seriously risk losing those gains.

In other words, those extra years of life thanks to antibiotics are not cemented into our lifespan. We live longer at the grace of these medications and if they disappear because of becoming ineffective, suddenly we'll be dying young again. Antimicrobial resistance on a global scale could make the COVID pandemic seem like a wee sniffle. On the downside, animal (mice) studies suggest that antibiotics early in life can change the microbiome to a more pro-ageing, inflammatory profile, which shortens lifespan. We'll never be sure that's true in humans but it does mean that after a course of antibiotics in both kids and adults, some attention to a diverse dietary pattern with some fermented foods might be a good idea.

Antibiotics may do more, though: Interestingly, most of our antibiotics started off as natural substances in bacteria, especially those which live in the soil. No-one's too sure why bacteria have their own antibiotics. It may be to protect themselves against attack by other micro-organisms, but natural antibiotics may also not be there to function as antibiotics at all. There is some laboratory evidence that they act on mitochondria – the energy sources in our cells which help to drive ageing – perhaps rejuvenating them. This is all the more fascinating since the evolutionary origins of mitochondria may be that they were once bacteria and over millions of years became incorporated into the cells of other organisms. Some antibiotics – again in the lab – may act a bit like rapamycin or resveratrol but clearly their effect on lifespans by treating infection and their threat to lifespan by messing with the microbiome likely overwhelms any benefit at the cellular level.

Antioxidant supplements?

#nup
#saveyourmoney

Sadly, despite oxidative stress being at the heart of ageing, antioxidant supplements like vitamins C and E and minerals like selenium have not been shown to make a dent in the diseases of ageing such as heart disease, cancer and dementia. If they did have an effect on ageing, you'd expect it to show up in reductions in the diseases it causes.

PART 6

It's not so bad to change what's on the outside

#dontbelievehype
#choosecarefully
#itcosts

Quick lift: The easiest way to change our appearance is through plastic surgery. It won't make you younger on the inside but might make you feel a lot better … if you can afford it, need it and choose the right surgeon. Me, I wouldn't go near anyone who hasn't trained and fully qualified as a plastic surgeon and, even then, shop around. Price is not an indication of quality and skill. Be very wary of having procedures when you're young. Once you've had an operation, there's no going back and since you haven't done anything about the underlying ageing process, depending on the surgery it's likely you'll need a re-do at some point, with added risks of complications each time. The later you start, the fewer the re-do's. The best plastic surgery is the surgery that no-one can tell you've had. They just say to you that you're looking great and assume you've had a holiday not realising that the holiday has been at home or in a hotel recovering for a week with a pressure helmet on.

The number of people undergoing plastic surgery has steadily risen since World War 1. Plastic surgery is most popular amongst women, who account globally for more than 80 per cent of all procedures. In the United States, there's been a huge spike in aesthetic surgery over the past 20 years. Cosmetic procedures are cheaper and more accessible now than before. A bit further into the section we'll unpack them with a non-judgemental guide for men and women.

It's important, though, to contextualise this desire to look younger.

Escaping the stigma of ageing or reinforcing it?

There is a lot of stigma associated with ageing, particularly towards women. Researchers from the Women's and Gender Studies Program and Sociology Department at Boston College claim that the idea of 'successful ageing' is linked to not *looking* old and therefore, they argue, actually promotes the stigmatisation of old age. Moreover, the notion that it's an individual's choice about how they age can increase the likelihood and blame ... and *shame* ... of 'allowing' yourself to look old. Other social researchers suggest that 'successful ageing' increasingly hints at a quest for *agelessness*. They write, 'For some, the seduction of agelessness merges with the seduction of technology – technology becomes a means-to-agelessness – with aged flesh being "whisked away" thereby "cheating mother nature".'

These researchers looked at whether the proliferation of procedures and technologies and associated marketing fuel demand and increase the pressure on women to continue to meet and comply with feminine beauty norms as they age. They ask, is it empowering, oppressive or both? Remember, of course, that this is a biased sample since you need money and the freedom to spend it to be in the market for plastic surgery.

Of the largely white middle-class American women who were studied, most liked the ready access to anti-ageing procedures. A 47-year-old woman expressed the comforting thought that she could whip out and 'fix' a problem. The conclusion was that ageing successfully, in light of the prevalence and availability of these procedures, comes to mean not only maintaining a healthy, active body through exercise and eating well, but a young-looking body (and face) through surgery or injectables like botox and fillers.

Is plastic surgery ageist or are we getting on our moral high horse?

Dr Bridget Garnham at the University of South Australia did some research in 2013 about the anti-ageing 'discourse' and the commonly held view that cosmetic surgery is, at heart, ageist.

The research hypothesised that aesthetic surgery is undertaken to look better, not younger, and that plastic surgery can be reimagined as 'self care', giving older people the freedom to look the way they choose. This allows people to experience their idea of 'older' while rejecting the tag of 'elderly'.

So, in this view, it's surgery to redesign 'older' rather than denying ageing.

Dr Garnham cites practitioners from the cosmetic surgery industry who have experience working with older patients. When they're asked about how the world at large views elderly people who want to change their appearance, these doctors and nurses say they hear words like 'disgusting' and cite younger people who say, 'Why do they bother?' The general opinion, they claim, is often of it being 'ick'.

In this sense, anti-ageing procedures do perhaps allow people to buck those stereotypes of old age. Away from our prejudices, these procedures may enable those fortunate enough to have the resources to live a life consistent with how we see ourselves, rather than the way our face looks.

There are important consumer issues, though ...

Choosing the surgeon or doctor

You make up your own mind on this. All I'll say is that there are large amounts of money to be made in plastic surgery, so there are lots of doctors who want to drink at the fountain. You'll find ENT surgeons who'll do a nose job, eye surgeons who'll do a lift around the eyes, gynaecologists who'll do labiaplasties, dermatologists who'll do a variety of procedures, and general practitioners who've done courses in cosmetic surgery who'll do all kinds of operations. At the time of writing, the regulators who are supposed to keep the public safe have done a pretty terrible job of that, which makes your choice tough.

My starting point is that plastic surgeons are trained to do this stuff and, yes, like all professional groups, there are good ones and not so good ones but at least they've done the hard yards. Take a face and neck lift, for example. Done properly it's a skilled and sometimes difficult operation which requires keyhole access, delicate reduction and stitching of the fragile layers of neck muscles under the chin and hidden scars around the ears. Yes, there are some ENT surgeons who are very good at reshaping the nose but if you need other plastic procedures then they aren't necessarily the right speciality to be seeing and good ENT surgeons will be the first to tell you that. Dermatologists and GPs are not trained surgeons and it takes years of training under supervision to know how to handle different tissues, what incisions are likely to give the best results, and the stitching that needs to be done for minimal scarring. So me, I'd instinctively avoid anyone who calls themselves a cosmetic physician or surgeon. You haven't a clue what you're getting. Some will tell you they've done hundreds of these operations and show you photographs but that could mean they're self-taught and photographs can be manipulated. Be very careful of anything near the eyes and you really need to be sure that anyone you use to operate in that area is properly trained. Some eye surgeons (ophthalmologists) have sub-specialised in eye plastics but you'd want to see where and when.

You need to talk to people who've been to a particular surgeon and ask them how it went. If your friends talk about the work they've had done, do you admire it or think, 'not in a month of Sundays'?

It's also really important to get an accurate idea of costs, including anaesthetist, theatre and hospital, and exactly what convalescence involves. For example, if you've had a face lift you'll need to be in a compression helmet for up to a week. Where are you going to spend that week if you don't want anyone to know that you've had stuff done?

Know what you want to achieve and why you're doing it

If you're a woman you may want to achieve the plumped-up Kardashian look and breasts which tell the world that you've had work done. If you're a bloke, you might want a washboard abdomen and a chiselled Brad Pitt jaw.

But do you really want people to know you've had plastic surgery?

This is an evolving story partly because of the rise of social media, especially in the lives of children and young adults. The pandemic saw many people looking at themselves on screens for hours a day, for months at a stretch. There's anecdotal evidence to support the idea that when restrictions lifted, people's first port of call was the injectables clinic. Very little research has been done on the correlation between social factors and individual thoughts and behaviour when it comes to our wanting to change our appearance, which is strange, really, when you consider the huge spike in the popularity of cosmetic surgery and easy access to procedures.

But social factors are *crucial* in this discussion and you need to be sure of what you're actually buying because once the scalpel has gone in, there's no going back.

I touched on this in my first book, *So You Think You Know What's Good For You?* When considering what happens to women in their 40s – after they've had children but before menopause – medical science needs to be supplemented by social science with its analysis of the complexity of relationships and expectations.

Do you want people to realise that your forehead looks smooth and your facial muscles aren't moving because you've had so much botox or that your lips are puckered or maximally pumped? Or pretend they didn't notice? Again, anecdotal evidence would tell you that people like being told they look 'fresh' and 'alert'.

A group of Australian researchers has found some qualitative evidence that plastic surgery recipients can be perceived negatively by others. Of a group of 20 women who'd had breast augmentations, many reported feeling stigmatised in that they were perceived by others as unstable and insecure. One husband was reported as saying, 'I don't want you to turn into this, you know, fake kind of thing.'

For what my view is worth, the best plastic surgery, as I said before, is the plastic surgery no-one recognises you've had, but elicits comments about how well you're looking and whether you've bought some new clothes. This is the sign of an expert surgeon who's done only just enough to achieve a good result but not so much that they might have stretched things too far and not allowed for future interventions.

Durability of plastic surgery

What happens to that tummy tuck you had in your 50s, when you're pushing 70?

Or the hair replacement surgery that you had during middle age that is now diminished as your skin loses its bounce?

Common sense will tell you that a breast enlargement in your young adult years will look different 30 years later. Breast augmentation surgery normally lasts about ten years before the implants have to be replaced. Face and neck lifts also have a time limit as the tissues age and continue to sag.

You've got to have the conversation with the specialist about their complication rates, what to expect (for example, a face lift takes a while to settle so looks better at the beginning than after a few weeks) and how long your $25,000 investment in your face will last (probably only ten years, maybe less). Everything changes as we age: muscles, tendons and bones. It's not just the skin, it's the architecture of what lies beneath. When it comes to a face lift, it might need to be repeated and won't do much for wrinkles, only sags. That's where botox and fillers come in. But a warning with botox: after using it, you may start to lose volume in your face and thus the process of ageing could be accelerated. Good botox clinics tend to use the smallest possible dose.

Researchers in Boston have looked at how frailty affects the outcome of the surgery, showing that wounds take longer to heal in older people.

A man thing

A Canadian study found that the notion of remaking the body via plastic surgery was associated with shifting notions of masculinity. In their study, in-depth interviews were conducted amongst men aged 18–53 who'd undergone surgery or were contemplating it.

All interviewees spoke about wanting to look more masculine. They wanted to look leaner and more muscular, often sportier. They knew about male celebrities like Brad Pitt or David Beckham.

The research revealed a paradox: many were comfortable with their own use of plastic surgery but not supportive of other men having the same procedures. Many associated it with homosexuality, or femininity, and a notion that it was 'too excessive' (even though they'd had work done themselves). Some men tried to couch it as a need, rather than a want. So when one man went in for a rhinoplasty and then consented to have more widespread aesthetic changes to his nose, he couched it as a medical procedure, rather than aesthetic surgery.

Most men saw the surgery as a way to exercise control over their bodies and increase their self-confidence. So plastic surgery has joined bodybuilding, tattooing and other mainstream body modification practices for men.

Men probably need to be even more careful about their choice of surgeon since their hairlines can make it harder to hide scars.

Everyone's doing it ... aren't they?

It's probably more widespread than you think. It's very easy to get some 'work done'. The notion of 'work' sits on a spectrum, of course. But if you want a quick forehead freeze, you can pop into a suburban clinic and be out in under an hour. Just be a sensible and careful buyer.

PART 7

While you're waiting on the magic pill of youth

Avoid the slow-moving cluster-f...

#dontwait
#nomagichere

Quick take: It's easy to lose sight of the obvious when you get into the weeds on what helps you to live younger longer. Don't get mugged by reality. Might be boring but do the basics no matter what chronological age you are. Smoking burnt plants, especially tobacco, high blood pressure, raised blood fats, lack of physical activity and being overweight or obese all speed up biological ageing. Sometimes it's by physical battering (blood pressure), sometimes it's toxins and sometimes it's an activated immune system which causes inflammation and tissue damage. So, if you can, attend to these risk factors rather than hoping some simple bottle of stuff in the pharmacy will do the job.

Quit smoking

A woman who smokes 20 per day at the age of 20 and doesn't quit is likely to die 14 years sooner than a woman who's never smoked, and the chances of premature death rise with the number of cigarettes smoked. On average, female never-smokers have a 9–14-year gain in life expectancy at age 20 compared to any current smoking females, and in males it's 7–10 years. If you're 70 and still smoke, you've only a 7 per cent chance of getting to 90. If you don't smoke then your chances could be as high as 33 per cent. In middle age, smoking doubles your chances of dying too soon. Quitting at age 40 restores men to the life expectancy they'd have had if they'd never smoked – in other words, about a ten-year gain. Quitting at 50 adds six years to your life and halves your chances of a fatal smoking-related event.

If you're a smoker, there's nothing you can buy online, in the pharmacy or put in your cooking pot that gains you so many years of healthy life as quitting or never smoking to start with. There's a long list of conditions which smoking causes and from which you die early and often miserably. These include cancer, heart disease, stroke, dementia and chronic obstructive lung disease. And if you think smoking weed is safer, it may well not be.

Smoking's also a classic example of how risk factors cluster. Smokers are more likely to be poor, have less education, be socially isolated, have other medical problems, work in more dangerous situations, drink alcohol excessively, take less exercise and not wear seatbelts. Smokers are also far more likely to have depression or a major mental illness like schizophrenia and use other substances. The bottom line is that for a lot of people just telling them to quit won't cut it. They need support. The other piece of information you need to have is that just cutting the number of cigarettes you smoke each day isn't enough. For reasons researchers don't fully understand, the first ten cigarettes are the most dangerous. So quitting means quitting.

Get that high blood pressure down

Biological ageing is speeded up by high blood pressure, which in turn sets up a cascade of events which can lead to an earlier grave than you might have planned. It's such a powerful risk factor for premature ageing that, arguably, you want to know what your blood pressure is from your 20s onwards and check it every few years. Raised blood pressure creeps up on you and can start when you're reasonably young, which is why every so often you should measure it at home or get your GP to check it during a visit. Measuring at home is often more accurate.

Here's the cascade

When your blood pressure is up, the pulse wave that comes out of your heart each time it beats physically batters your arteries, prematurely ageing and stiffening them. Stiffened arteries then increase your blood pressure even more because they resist the pressure wave coming out of your heart each time it contracts. High blood pressure also often goes along with carrying too much weight around your abdomen, which triggers your immune system, which then means the battering is accompanied by inflammation in your artery walls, which then means that whatever bad cholesterol (LDL) is circulating in your blood can more easily enter the now fragile internal walls of your arteries, causing scarring and a proneness to clotting. Stiff and narrowed arteries mean that vital organs receive less blood supply.

This is a slow-moving cluster-f... which gathers speed if you don't put the brakes on and try getting into reverse. It's an insidious combination which makes your heart and brain ancient before their time, and makes you prone to heart attacks, heart failure, strokes, kidney damage, glaucoma and dementia.

'Hypertension' is the technical term for high blood pressure but it's misleading and can make you think that stress is the cause. While chronic stress is linked to high blood pressure, it's far from the only factor. Others include family history, smoking, overweight, high salt intake, too much alcohol and kidney damage, which is commoner than you think. Coming back to chronic stress (see Does the Mind Matter?), it could be from, say, having a job where your boss orders you around and doesn't give you much chance to decide how to do the job or set your own priorities, or from poverty and social dislocation. That kind of pressure does raise the level of stress hormones – adrenaline and noradrenaline – and fires up the sympathetic nervous system, the network of nerves that prepares the body for emergencies by, among other things, constricting arteries and raising blood pressure. So psychological stresses are not to be ignored but solely focusing on them is a mistake because there's a lot more going on.

Arterial stiffness is another measure of biological ageing. The stiffer your vessels, the older you are internally. A measure of this is a larger than average gap between the systolic and diastolic blood pressures (top and bottom numbers). For example, you might have a blood pressure of 165/85 mmHg. This is called a raised pulse pressure. Moderate intensity exercise on most days of the week helps to keep your arteries nice and elastic.

So what's the blood pressure level that helps keep you young?

Well, that depends on what else is going on in your body. If you're healthy with no other problems, the official level is 120/80. But that's almost certainly not the blood pressure we evolved to live with. Hunter-gatherers often have lower blood pressures because of exercise and low salt intake and some studies suggest that increased risk starts when the top figure rises above 115. If you've had heart disease, a stroke or diabetes, then the evidence is that you should aim to get your blood pressure a bit lower than what they call normal.

Get cuffed: Now, while measuring your blood pressure might seem straightforward, it's not. You shouldn't have taken any caffeinated drinks or smoked for a couple of hours beforehand. You need to have been relaxed and settled for a while and your blood pressure should be measured twice in the same arm with a cuff that's big enough for the size of your arm. If the pressure's high at your doctor's, there's about a 30 per cent chance it'll be significantly lower at home. If you do take readings at home, it's increasingly thought that a blood pressure which is up at night is a sign of hypertension.

What can be done?

If your blood pressure is up, you need to see your doctor and get it sorted out. There are quite a few things you can do to avoid it rising as you age and help get it down if it's up:

Lose weight: 10 per cent weight loss can be the equivalent of a blood pressure pill.

Exercise at moderate intensity most days of the week: This can also achieve a similar blood pressure reduction to a medication.

Cut your alcohol intake: This can produce a significant lowering if your blood pressure is high.

Reduce your salt intake (see Cut the Salt): This can have an immediate effect and also helps avoid a rise in blood pressure as you get older.

Chronic stress reduction: Not always an easy thing to do.

Your kidneys count

This is another cluster-f… in the making. The things that age us biologically often damage our kidneys as well. In turn, chronic kidney damage speeds up ageing and is associated in particular with increased risks of heart attacks and strokes and dying younger than you should. The trouble is that by the time one of the standard tests of kidney function – the creatinine level in your blood – is registering as abnormal, you've already lost 30–40 per cent of your kidney function. A more sensitive test is the eGFR, which is an indication of how well your kidneys are filtering waste products (one of which is, in fact, creatinine). Most pathology labs in Australia include eGFR in their reports. Another test is cystatin-C and while this is not routinely carried out, some researchers believe it is better than either creatinine or eGFR testing.

Keeping your kidneys young: Having a mother who was healthy and didn't smoke or have high blood pressure during pregnancy is a good start, because poor maternal health can lead to a baby with smaller kidneys and therefore less reserve for the future. That said, you can't go back and fix that for yourself, but what you can do is keep your blood pressure low by losing weight, exercising, limiting salt and alcohol intake or taking medications if necessary, not smoking, possibly avoiding advanced glycation end products (AGEs) and following a Mediterranean-style diet.

Get that fat right out of your blood

#goodbadandugly

Quick points: Be sure your blood fat (lipid) tests are accurate. If they come back raised, it may be worth repeating them to double-check. Focus on HDL (good), LDL (bad), total cholesterol (a mix of the good and the bad) and triglycerides (bad). Even if your risk profile is good, aim low with LDL and triglycerides and aim high-ish with HDL. Triglycerides are important, not least because they can make your LDL cholesterol more toxic. Raising HDL by natural means, such as exercise and weight loss, is best since artificial ways of doing it through drugs or infusions have not worked so far for reasons which are yet to be properly explained. Follow the Mediterranean-style dietary pattern. Plant sterols in margarine do work. Eat oily fish once or twice a week and don't waste your money or the environment on fish oil supplements. If your overall risk profile isn't good, especially if you have diabetes or the metabolic syndrome, get your LDL as low as possible and make sure your triglycerides aren't raised. Keep your waist circumference at or below the recommended size. If your cholesterol levels are really high, then that could mean you have a genetic issue which needs to be diagnosed and treated with a degree of urgency. However, for most people who have modestly raised lipids, whether you need medications depends on your total risk rather than just the levels themselves. Know your total risk by doing a risk score: see http://www.cvdcheck.org.au/

Step one is knowing while you're still young what your blood fat (lipid) levels are. If you're aged around 20 with a low cholesterol and things stay that way, you can live up to nine years longer than a 20-year-old with high levels who doesn't do anything about them. However, just having a high *total* cholesterol may be too crude a measure of risk. You really need to go deeper and know your levels of HDL, LDL and triglycerides. There's an argument to be made that if your lipids are raised, you should have a second test just to be sure.

In the family? At any age, if your total cholesterol is really high (7.5 mmol/L or more) or you've got an LDL that's 5 mmol/L or more, it can mean you have a genetic problem called familial hypercholesterolaemia which needs to be treated actively and soon. The likelihood of this is increased if you have family members who developed heart disease relatively young (under 55 in men and under 60 in women).

Most of us don't get to those levels. For us, it's the way we eat and live that's the main influence on our cholesterol and, to understand your risk, it's not enough just to measure your blood lipids. You need to know what's called your 'absolute risk score', based on a combination of factors including blood pressure and your age. A lot of this, though, depends on your age and most absolute risk scores don't work when you're younger. When you're young, it's important to know whether there's an issue with blood pressure or lipids so you can change your diet or your intake of alcohol and inhaled burnt plants, as well as physical activity levels.

Back to lipids.

HDL (high density lipoprotein) is the good stuff and helps to remove cholesterol from your arteries. For every mmol/L (millimoles per litre) your HDL goes up, your risk of a heart attack or other cardiac event goes down. There is a limit, however, because very high levels of HDL can increase your heart risk, which means you should only use natural ways to raise it, such as exercise, weight loss, quitting cigarettes, keeping alcohol intake low, reducing your saturated fat intake and increasing the monounsaturated fats. Statins don't do much for your HDL. They're aimed at LDL. Older drugs like niacin and fibrates raise HDL to some extent but they have side effects.

LDL (low density lipoprotein) is the nasty one. It carries cholesterol inside the walls of your arteries then gets oxidised (biological rusting) by an inflamed immune system from an unhealthy lifestyle and possibly a microbiome that fires up inflammation rather than dampening it. This process forms the basis of atherosclerosis, which narrows the artery and which can break open and allow a clot to form, causing a heart attack or stroke depending on which artery is involved. The simplest message is that you should keep your LDL as low as you can. Some cardiologists measure 'very low density lipoprotein' cholesterol (VLDL) because they believe it's a better marker of risk than LDL. There isn't much convincing evidence that in most people it's any better than your triglyceride level. That's because VLDL contains a lot of triglyceride and when you lower your triglycerides the VLDL seems to follow. Refined carbohydrates like sugar are bad for VLDL levels and could explain why sugar intake is associated with an increased risk of heart attacks and strokes.

Triglycerides: These are probably undervalued as a risk factor, which is a shame since they're very sensitive to lifestyle changes and can be a problem, especially in women. High triglyceride levels make your LDL even more toxic. In men, for every 1 mmol/L rise in triglycerides, there's a 14 per cent rise in the risk of heart attacks and other coronary problems, whereas in women the increase is 37 per cent. These risks rise with age.

Triglycerides can be seen best in meat. The visible fat is full of them.

Levels of triglycerides go up with excessive alcohol, some medications like steroids and the contraceptive pill, abdominal fat, pre-diabetes and diabetes, kidney damage and autoimmune diseases like SLE (lupus).

It's often quite easy to reduce your triglycerides with lifestyle changes like weight loss, reducing unhealthy fats in your diet and increasing exercise. There are medications but that needs a discussion with your GP.

Fish oil and staying young and alive? Nup. Not much evidence at all for that despite huge numbers of people swallowing fish oil capsules every day. The confusion arises from earlier studies which, although they seemed to suggest that fish oil prevented cardiac deaths, were too small and poorly designed. As larger, better studies have been done, sadly the much touted benefits of fish oil supplements have largely disappeared at least when it comes to saving or prolonging lives. Much better eating whole fish as a red meat replacement in your diet.

Your abdomen and staying young

Top line numbers: Caucasian men should be aiming for a waist circumference of 94 cm or less, and for women 80 cm or less. If you're ethnically Chinese or Asian-Indian, then the target for women is the same but men should aim lower, at less than 89 cm. Basically, if you're male, regardless of your race, if you take a size 34 in jeans then you're significantly more likely to be in better shape and have a longer life than the guy next to you at the rack who's trying on a size 40. In terms of what it means in years lost and gained: if you're an overweight (BMI 25–29.9) non-smoker, you lose three years off your life on average. If you're an obese (BMI 30 and over) non-smoking woman, you can expect to lose seven years off your life and, in that shorter life, more years will be spent in ill health. Obese men live on average six years less and, on top of that, experience even more time in illness before they die than obese women. Obese smokers lose about twice as many years. If you have the metabolic syndrome (see You Don't Need the Metabolic Syndrome in Your Life) then compared to people who don't have it, you've triple the chances of having a heart attack or stroke, double the chances of dying of one, and five times the chances of developing type 2 diabetes. The problem begins in your 20s if not earlier but can be stopped.

Focus on your waist: Your visceral fat, the fat inside your abdomen, is pretty toxic. It's metabolically active, meaning that the unhealthy fats in tummy storage can be easily taken out of stock and put into the bloodstream. Visceral fat activates inflammation and resists insulin, the hormone which takes sugar (glucose) out of your blood and puts it into cells. Insulin resistance is at the core of type 2 diabetes for a couple of reasons. One is the rise in blood glucose, which is toxic in its own right. The other is that a high insulin level has metabolic effects itself. Some experts think that, on the other hand, subcutaneous fat is not particularly dangerous. The biggest growth in waist circumference tends to happen in a person's 50s and is more common in men. It can actually happen without overall weight gain, so the tightness of your clothes might be a better indicator than the scales. This goes to being aware of your metabolic shape – literally – as you get into your late 30s and 40s and beyond. The changes are slow and insidious. A few hundred grams here and there soon become kilos. But while weight gain might be under the radar, having trouble getting into clothes is an amber light, particularly when you can't button up that blouse, shirt or jacket. I'm lucky. I have the regular humiliation of having to find a jacket I can button for television stand-ups. Nothing like it to motivate a return to dietary restriction.

Fatness measures

BMI: A body mass index of 30 or more is the definition of obesity, whereas overweight is defined as a BMI between 25 and 29.9. You calculate your BMI by dividing your weight in kilograms by your height in metres squared.

Waist circumference: Get a tape measure. Stand up. Take off your top; loosen your pants or skirt; feel for the highest point on your hip bone at the side of your waist (the iliac crest); then feel for the lower edge of your ribs just above the hip bone. You circle your tape measure approximately at the midpoint between the two. Breathe out and make sure the tape measure is snugly around you but not tight. At this point, you're allowed to cheat. You should find the smallest circumference just above or below the midpoint and take that as your waist circumference. Either way, it doesn't really matter as long as you always use the same technique.

Waist to hip ratio (WHR): It's a good indicator of heart and stroke risk but has its problems. It's calculated by dividing your waist measurement by the widest circumference around your buttocks. WHR should probably be 0.9 or less in men and 0.8 or less in women. The trouble with WHR is that a person who's 20 and thin might have a good looking WHR of less than 0.8. They might then put on weight around both their hips and abdomen. It's possible that their BMI goes into the obese range while the waist to hip ratio has stayed the same, even though the waist circumference has gone from a 26 to a 36 (i.e. into the risk zone).

So what's best?

#mirrormirroronthewall

For staying younger longer, it's your waist circumference. Although, unless you're all muscle, if you have a BMI of over 30, the news is not good. And don't delude yourself in front of the mirror that you're a muscle machine when you know you're not. In many people, waist expansion is the first event which leads to a progressive elevation in blood pressure, blood fats and your level of blood sugar when you're fasting. That's the metabolic syndrome – a real life-shortener.

You don't need the metabolic syndrome in your life

It predicts diabetes, having a heart attack or a stroke, or all three. Compared to people who don't have the metabolic syndrome, you've triple the chances of having a heart attack or stroke, double the chances of dying of one, and five times the chances of developing type 2 diabetes.

To score a diagnosis, you need three out of the five criteria below based on European and Australian definitions of a healthy waist circumference, which depends on your ethnicity because some groups are more sensitive to abdominal fat:

* Europeans (Caucasians), people from the Middle East and Eastern Mediterranean, and probably Sub-Saharan Africans – men 94 cm or more; women 80 cm or more
* Japanese, Chinese, Indian, Pakistani, other Asian, Central and South American and probably Indigenous people – men 85–90 cm or more; women 80 cm or more
* A high triglyceride level of 1.7 mmol/L or more; a low HDL cholesterol of 1.03 mmol/L or less in men and 1.29 mmol/L or less in women
* A high blood pressure of 130/85 or more on the top or bottom number
* A fasting blood sugar that's 5.6 mmol/L or more

Reversing the damage: Weight loss of even just 5 or 10 per cent can make a big difference and changes to exercise levels and diet can bring down the other factors. You also need to talk to your GP about whether metformin might be merited if you're just on the edge of diabetes. Metformin, to remind you, is an inexpensive anti-diabetic medication which can help with weight loss and may have anti-ageing effects (see Which Pill and Why?).

Losing fat: Learn to like being hungry and to do that you've got to become hungry first. So (and this is going to shock you) eat less. Know what carb and protein sizes truly are and what you should have each day.

Portions: For example, one carbohydrate portion of cooked rice is about half a cup, and for dinner you probably shouldn't be having more than three carb portions in total. If you can afford it, a sensible dietician will help you with a plan.

Weigh yourself daily after your shower in the morning. Accept that it will vary and that a bad weekend may not show up on Monday morning because you might have been in calorie deficit and it'll take a while to flow through. As night follows day, eating too much will eventually appear on the scales.

Keep an honest daily food diary when you're trying to lose weight. There are a few good apps for this. Only eat what's put in front of you. No hoovering off the kids' or partner's plates. Eat most of your calories during the day when you have a chance to burn some of them off. Don't change your diet at weekends.

Exercise: Aim for an hour of real exercise a day.

What about sex?

#yes
#duuuh

Not as much evidence as you'd think: A British study of men over two decades found that having sex twice or more per week was associated with reduced chances of dying from coronary heart disease. This could be the sex (that's my view) or because to have sex frequently you need to be fairly fit. Another small study found that women who'd enjoyed sex during their lives lived longer. No pressure.

When you think about it, sex brings together a lot of things that are important for living younger longer. It is (well, should be) about intimacy, relationships, social contact, fitness and hopefully life satisfaction. As I discussed at length in *So You Think You Know What's Good For You?*, too many people in

LGBTIQ communities who need freedom and flexibility to express their gender identity find themselves struggling with stigma imposed on them and the search for satisfying sexual and personal relationships. This can and does create inordinate psychological distress and we all share responsibility for reducing stigma and creating a community that's more permissive to people's identities.

Staying young is orchestral

#getthebastardsbackintune
#thesumoftheparts
#bewarethehockeystick

If you read my last book, you may recall that risk factors hunt in packs. Strokes, heart attacks and cancers are usually caused by a combination of raised blood pressure and lipids (sometimes by not very much), sluggish sugar metabolism due to insulin resistance due to physical inactivity, weak muscles and visceral fat, fuelled by a crap diet that's too low in vegetables, lacks diversity and consequently creates a pro-ageing microbiome, plus maybe some inherited genes in the background, not to mention air pollution, too much sun, avoidable viral infections (hepatitis B, HIV, HPV) and chronic stress. Even unsafe sex gets a look in, and I haven't even mentioned smoking burnt plants, the worst of all. When it comes to maths, these factors don't know about addition or subtraction or indeed graphs that go up in a steady line. The mathematics of risk factors is based on multiplication, not addition, which means the graphs can go up really steeply when the levels of these factors are quite low.

False self-reassurance that things don't look too bad can be deadly because these variables feed on each other and create what is, in fact, an epidemic curve inside your body. The good news about the deadly multiplication story is that reducing as many factors as you can gets you a lot more than simple subtraction.

The prize for changing what you can is high. Strokes account for roughly one in ten deaths and a lot of miserable years with disability. Heart disease takes about one in six lives and many unhappy years before that. Cancer and dementia take the rest.

The jargon term for effective prevention of toxic ageing is 'multiple risk factor reduction'. When you're young (let's say, under 50) with no strong family history of people dying or being diagnosed young from cancer or heart disease, you achieve multiple risk factor reduction by dietary pattern, occasional dietary frugality, daily moderate to intense exercise, not smoking, safe sex, immunisation, cervical cancer screening and sun avoidance. If you've a family history of early heart disease or cancer, you may need far more intense surveillance following genetic counselling. (See Get Out of Those Genes.)

Once you're 50, add regular screening for breast and bowel cancer, and round about that age it's probably worth checking what's called your 'absolute risk score' in case your lifestyle needs a bit of help from a medication for cholesterol or blood pressure reduction.

Foretelling the future: There are tools around which try to predict your future – at least five or ten years out – but most are limited to heart disease, diabetes and stroke. Common variables which are plugged into these tools for heart disease predictions are age, gender, total cholesterol, HDL cholesterol, whether you smoke, your systolic blood pressure (that's the top number) and whether you're on treatment for high blood pressure. But they leave a lot out. For instance, while depression might be as strong a risk factor for coronary heart disease as cholesterol, most predictive tools don't take that into account. Central adiposity (your waist circumference) is important for the risk of heart disease and type 2 diabetes and, again, many tools miss that out. Exercise makes a big difference to survival and some argue that going from sedentary to active is at least as good for your health as quitting smoking, yet exercise isn't in many equations. There's also debate about the impact of blood tests for inflammation (C reactive protein, CRP, is one of these) in risk assessment tools. What I'm saying is that the risk tools are important but so is what they leave out in terms of taking personal action.

Another word on inflammation: I've mentioned it several times so far. It's an add-on to the free radical and oxidation story because inflammation can speed up tissue damage and ageing. It is also an essential enabler of cholesterol damage to artery walls causing atherosclerosis, narrowing and potential blockage if a clot forms. To make things worse, inflammation makes the blood more prone to clotting, and these damaged arteries more twitchy and liable to heart attack–inducing spasm.

For some reason yet to be discovered, anti-inflammatory drugs don't influence this much and antioxidant vitamins either don't help or may make it worse. Daily low dose aspirin is really only of value if you've already had a heart attack, stroke or cardiac problem like angina. The good news is that inflammation does respond to the stay-young changes I've been talking about throughout the book.

Don't be beguiled by the word 'normal': There's no such thing as normal. Most risk factors (apart from smoking, alcohol and other drugs) are on a sliding scale from low to high, and groups of experts – sometimes compromised by payments from the pharmaceutical industry – have drawn a line where they think normal lies and above which you're in disease territory. The reason for mentioning the drug industry is that if you draw the line low, then more people might qualify for medications that they may not need. What your personal aim should be is to get your levels down to the low side of the scale. With smoking there's no low side – only stopping altogether because the most dangerous cigarettes are the first ten. If you have a drug and alcohol problem, then stopping might be your only option.

Cut the salt

#saltyenoughalready

The sprinkle: Of all the deaths from heart disease, excess salt intake is a significant cause in more than 1.5 million of them each year. Salt raises blood pressure and makes the natural increase of blood pressure with age worse and, as a consequence, the risks of stroke and heart attacks go up. Salt may also increase oxidative stress and inflammation and the risk of Alzheimer's disease and autoimmune diseases like rheumatoid arthritis. Most salt comes from processed foods rather than the salt you add. Making flavoursome, herb-dense meals distracts from needing added salt. Reducing how much food you eat through portion control will reduce your salt intake without you having to think much about it.

Know how much salt you're eating: There are two measures: sodium and salt. Sodium is what does the damage but it comes in salt, which is sodium chloride, and salt weighs 2.5 times more than its sodium content. The aim should be to keep your sodium intake to 2 g a day. That's 5 g of salt. So if the pack says there's 500 mg of salt in a serving, that's 200 mg of sodium, which is 10 per cent of your target intake. Five grams of salt is about a teaspoonful. Australian men eat double the recommended intake for them, and women 50 per cent more. Men are consuming over 10 g of salt a day and women well over 7 g. That's a lot of extra sodium a day and mostly from processed foods including bread. Salt increases your blood pressure and your risk of heart attacks and strokes in various ways. Too much sodium in the blood makes your kidneys retain more water and that raises blood pressure. It's also pretty clear that excess sodium can damage arteries in its own right and is linked to stiffer, less elastic arteries, which in turn can make high blood pressure worse, as well as the kidney damage it causes. High blood pressure and diabetes are the commonest causes of kidney damage as people age and kidney damage adds to the risk of premature death from heart disease.

The damage that salt can do to arteries – particularly the lining (endothelium) – could be behind the observation that salt intake is related to the risk of Alzheimer's disease. Experiments in mice have shown that dietary salt can induce the production of the tau protein, which gums up the brains of people with cognitive decline and Alzheimer's. One possibility is that salt increases oxidative stress in the memory part of the brain called the hippocampus. This oxidative stress may also increase the chances of cholesterol damaging the arteries through atherosclerosis. Excessive salt intake is moderately associated with the risk of stomach (gastric) cancer in many studies. Salt may make the effects of the ulcer germ, *H. pylori*, worse and probably damages the stomach lining directly. There is growing evidence of a link between salt intake and autoimmune diseases such as rheumatoid arthritis and perhaps multiple sclerosis. The suggestion is that excessive sodium takes the foot off the brake which stops the immune system becoming inflamed and attacking various parts of the body, such as the linings of the joints (rheumatoid) and nerves (MS).

A weight loss or weight maintenance diet with portion control will lower sodium intake just because you're eating less. Cooking your own food rather than buying processed foods will help because you will be in control of the added salt. There is also evidence that you can fool your tastebuds by aromas from herbs, adding lemon juice to salads or cooked vegetables, using coarse pepper and even tiny amounts of ham.

Putting a lid on alcohol

#takecare
#smallmeanssmall

Alcohol is the leading cause of premature death and lost years of health in people aged 15–49. If you think you're drinking for your health, you're mostly deluded. Enjoy alcohol for its taste and as a social lubricant but don't ever think it's benign.

Moderate amounts in people with heart problems probably do help the heart a little through effects on HDL, but it's a fine line which has to be balanced against the risks of injury, violence, raised blood pressure, breast cancer and all the other problems alcohol use can bring. The trouble is that we tend to think that if a little is okay, more might be better; and if we assume that moderate use is healthy (albeit for one thing only – your heart) then our total consumption will drift upwards.

The good news is that small amounts of alcohol are not particularly harmful, assuming you're not pregnant or trying to conceive, you don't drive or do anything requiring skill afterwards, don't mix alcohol with other drugs – and you aren't obese. If you're obese, you've almost certainly got excess fat in your liver which is putting you on the path to serious liver damage. Every drink you have has a significantly increased risk of accelerating that liver damage, which could lead to cirrhosis.

What's small? Learn what a standard drink is. It's much less than you think. The advice from the National Health and Medical Research Council is no more than ten standard drinks a week and no more than four standard drinks in any day. That's if you're otherwise healthy. As I said, the risks go up the more fat you're carrying. The other factor is your age. Alcohol becomes a heightened problem the older you are because there's less brain and body reserve. While young people are drinking less, over 55-year-olds are too often drinking too much … no doubt to the consternation of their abstemious kids.

PART 8

Does the mind matter?

From the helicopter: Your brain, mind and body are a single entity. Inseparable. And the whole staying young thing starts in the brain. While we might romanticise about the mind, in fact the brain and the bits and pieces below the neck are all one and hugely interconnected. The brain, through our eyes, ears and skin and the immune systems in our gut and lungs, monitors the physical and social environments in which we live, and allows us to adapt mentally and physically, both consciously and unconsciously. If it's hot we sweat. If it's cold we shiver. Some men would argue that if we have gas, we fart and have no control over it. If the air is polluted, we cough and try to get rid of the garbage we're inhaling. If we have a crap boss who's on our tails the whole time and makes life miserable, our brain and body start to shift towards an 'always-on' hormonal battering ram, which wears us away. Poverty, dispossession and abuse can do that too. Life is a massive balancing act from the molecules inside our cells, to our heart and arteries, to our immune system, our digestive system, our lungs, our kidneys and our brains. This set of balances, as you now well know, is called homeostasis. Give our bodies a bit of a push, then like a punching bag clown, our body bounces back upright, ready for the next punch. Too many punches, the bag starts to lean at an angle, and later it might deflate entirely. The battering has shifted the balance – the homeostasis – and that's how we lose our youth. Our brain, mind and psychological state are intimately wrapped up in this whole balance thing and, for many people, that's where accelerated ageing starts, even though they might not realise it.

One: This is the word to keep in your head when you read what follows and I can't say it often enough. If our brain was situated inside our abdomen, rather than perched on our necks, then we'd probably have less trouble with the idea that the brain and mind are part of our body and fully integrated with it. We have one body, yet while that's the bleeding obvious, we often behave as if we have two bodies – one above the neck and the other below (and in the case of men, three bodies because there's clearly stuff that goes on below the waist which seems to have a mind of its own). Anyway, it's all one and some experts argue that the physical processes which age us, no matter whether we're 30, 50 or 70, start at the top and work their way down. The brain part of our body can help to keep us physically young or drive us to a premature crumble. We resent doctors who tell us or imply that our pain or tiredness is affected by our psychological state because we assume they're saying that our physical symptoms are all in our head and therefore either imaginary or caused by a mental health issue. That's not what the doctor is usually saying, however clumsily it might come out. Good clinicians, whether they be doctors, physios or nurses, know that they can fix a lot of stuff physically but still fail to make a patient feel better because the clinician hasn't dealt with that person's story; how they are in the world, their mood, their relationships, their work or the lack of it, their anxieties about money and fear of the future or the uncertainty of being that we all have to cope with. If our brain was nestled in amongst our bowels or next to the heart in our chest, I suspect we wouldn't react so strongly against the idea that our physical symptoms have anything to do with our minds and so it is with staying physically young and slowing ageing. It's easy to assume it's all about diet and exercise, when they're just part of the story. Our brains can drive physical ageing profoundly and there are two concepts you might find useful before we go on.

1. Stuff happens without us knowing it: Again, this is the bleeding obvious when you think about it but is worth emphasising. Our body mostly works below our level of consciousness, far beneath what our mind normally perceives. We're unconscious of pretty much everything that keeps us going, from breathing to blood circulation, to digestion, to fluid balance, to how our cells work, divide and renew themselves. To influence ageing, we've got to influence these subterranean processes and most of them are controlled to some extent by the brain.

2. The outside world becomes our inside world often via the brain: It's easy to understand our relationship with our environment when you think about viruses hovering in the air and infecting us via the nose and throat, when we catch gastro from unhygienic food preparation, when we eat a lousy diet and damage our microbiome, or when we breathe dirty air. The thing is that our bodies have to be exquisitely tuned to our environment to survive. The prize for missing a serious threat could be more rapid loss of our youth, and death before our time has come. Many of these threats are actually social, meaning they arise from the way we live, work and interact with others. We evolved as hunter-gatherers and while some 'wellness' writers have romanticised the Stone Age, hunter-gatherers survived by recognising risky situations and responding to them quickly and effectively.

Imagine you're in the Palaeolithic era, walking with your family group through the savannah grassland on a warm spring day. A gentle breeze is blowing and the grass is rustling. What do you think has more survival advantage: saying to your partner, 'Darling, what a beautiful day, so wonderful to hear the grass in the wind and smell the scent of the flowers, isn't it?' or 'Shit, grab the kids and run, sounds as though there's a tiger in the grass! I'll try to get him with my spear.' Social and psychological stress are not unique to our times. The Stone Age and the early agriculture periods were more stressful than you might imagine. There were conflicts over resources, family integrity and even which gods we believed in. There's no survival advantage to minimising real threats. We're tuned to fighting and flighting or bickering and bolting and while we've benefited from millions of years of evolution to have respiratory, digestive and immune systems which can cope with infections, toxins and a variety of foods, our biggest advantage has been our brains, which allowed us to adapt to new or unexpected circumstances. Sometimes, though, an adaptation that suited an acute circumstance – like a tiger in the grass or even the occasional family argument – isn't well designed for stuff that's ongoing. The same adaptation that may have saved our life in the Stone Age could actually make us age faster in the 21st century.

The slope that's not slippery enough

#thecontrolthing
#hilltoclimb
#understandinggaps

The gap in life expectancy and rates of heart disease, cancer, dementia, distress, despair and premature death is like a hill where some people get stuck at the bottom or somewhere on the slope while others are comfortably at the summit. When working out what causes this hill of life and death, the first thing many think about is wealth. Having money certainly helps people live longer than the poor and disadvantaged, but it's more than dollars. Wealthier people live in suburbs with cleaner air, better schools, shops selling healthier food, and more social infrastructure. They're often also suburbs that are more walkable.

Large studies have pinned down another very important factor and it goes to the mind mattering. Psychologists call it 'locus of control' and it's been adapted to something called 'job strain'. It's about how much pressure you feel under at work to perform and how much freedom – or latitude – you feel you have to decide how best to achieve the targets being set for you. Job strain has its equivalent in life, particularly if you're poor and pressed by circumstances. A healthy locus of control is where you feel you have agency over your life rather than it being determined by others or circumstances. An unhealthy locus of control raises the risk that you lose decision-making and planning capacity because you feel so powerless.

This is one of the causes of chronic stress and the disruption of homeostasis which can lead to ageing.

Kids and the punching bag clown

The punching bag may start to tilt in childhood: This is probably the starkest example of how brains respond to the external environment and how that response affects the rest of our bodies, sometimes for good and sometimes for ill. Politicians like nothing better than images of themselves at a primary school, a kindergarten or cuddling a baby at the shopping mall. They bang on about the importance of childhood and education yet refuse to fund early childhood education adequately. The factors that tilt the punching bag include poverty, unemployment, abuse, neglect, poor intellectual stimulation, separation from parents at a young age and housing insecurity. There's considerable evidence that family stress and maternal stress, in particular, affect unborn babies and can significantly reset the control of chronic stress in young children, which then in turn can affect the rest of the body. For example, mother and child stress can shorten a child's telomeres, not to mention the mother's. Telomeres are the structures at the end of chromosomes which act like a lifespan clock. Researchers believe that, in general, the longer your telomeres, the longer your healthy lifespan; and the shorter they are, the more chronic diseases you're likely to have and the earlier you may actually die. What also seems to happen is that your genes change the way they work. These are not mutations in the DNA itself. The shape and function of the genetic code change because of chemical reactions between parts of the famous double helix. It's called 'DNA methylation' and the name for the phenomenon is 'epigenetics'. In fact, DNA methylation is thought to be yet another timer which separates our biological age – our body's physical and functional age – from the number of years we have on the clock if we just go by birthdays. What's happening to these kids, and it happens to adults too, is effectively a brain-drain from the constant effort to cope with and adapt to adversity, trauma and repeated stress.

The brain-drain thing

How the brain-drain thing works: We have multiple ways of sensing our environment and almost all of these pass through the brain without our being aware of it. It's homeostasis – a balancing act – of enormous complexity. Our eyes, ears, skin, the microbiome in our gut and respiratory tract, and our immune system are all highly tuned to threats from the outside world. As an aside, we tend to think of our gut and airways as being inside our bodies when, in fact, they are outside surfaces open to the world. Things have to pass through the walls of these tubes into our bloodstream before they are truly inside us.

Back to the brain. You can skip the next couple of paragraphs if you can't be bothered with the technical detail and are happy to trust me when I say that a repeatedly stressful environment can profoundly change the way the brain and the rest of the body work, both in terms of our behaviour and the physical processes which can either keep us young and healthy or speed up the damage that makes us age.

Most organisms, from viruses to humans, at their most basic level are programmed for survival: to live and reproduce rather than die and become extinct. The COVID-19 virus, for example, does this without a brain but has a set of genes which are focused on how to infect us, get inside our body and tell it to produce thousands of copies of itself then be exhaled or coughed out so the process can start all over again in a new person. While human beings have more interesting, complex lives than viruses, we haven't lost that primitive drive to survive. Our brains are primarily designed for survival and adaptation to adverse circumstances. That adaptation to threats and the flexibility that goes with it are among the main reasons for our success as a species. Thinking, memory, learning, planning and decision-making, and their tight two-way links to the rest of the body such as the heart, lungs, immune system, kidneys and gut, make us formidable survivors. This integrated process is called 'allostasis'. But allostasis has a weakness. It's designed for intermittent threats and stress from the environment.

Some stress is good for us. We need it to enhance our performance, including learning, but if our interaction with our environment is relentlessly stressful – say, through lack of educational opportunities, a lousy job, not having enough money, relationship issues and in the case of First Nations peoples, displacement, dispossession, deprivation and alienation – things start to go awry. The parts of the brain which save us – like the hippocampus (memory), the amygdala (emotion and learning) and the prefrontal cortex (planning, decision-making and impulse control) – can start to work poorly, in a less coordinated way, and that in turn affects our ability to deal with new stresses and bounce back from them.

The question that often arises is why one person reacts to such stress badly and another sails through? The answer isn't known but is thought to relate to how much trauma and disruption a person has had, which may affect how they perceive the stresses they're exposed to. Some people may have genes that allow them to respond to stress in a less physical way. In the end, it's as much about how we perceive the demands being made of us as the demands themselves. Government policies that affect our social environment can mess with our allostasis. Disrupted allostasis from life experiences – such as where you see yourself in the social hierarchy and feelings of relative inequality, low income, poor education, an unsatisfying, unstable job and insecure housing – increases your likelihood of unhealthy behaviours, sickness and dying prematurely.

Here's just one example of how what goes on in the brain can reset your body in bad ways. Hormones are chemical messengers which travel through our blood and pass messages to different parts of the body. Some hormones get a woman ready for pregnancy each month or instruct a man's testes to produce sperm. Other hormones get our heart and arteries ready for an emergency, and may also put our thinking and memory into overdrive. Several of these hormone systems rely on the brain to control them, and what tends to happen is that one part of the brain tells another part what or what not to release into the bloodstream to tell an organ below the neck how it should behave. The classic example of this is called the hypothalamic-pituitary-adrenal (HPA) axis. The hypothalamus is very integrated into what's going on in the rest of the brain, while the pituitary is a tiny gland suspended beneath the brain, which produces an amazing range of messengers, often under instruction from the hypothalamus. One of the targets of the pituitary hormones are the adrenal glands, which sit on top of each kidney and, among other things, produce stress-related hormones such as cortisol, which in turn can affect our behaviour and the way the brain works. You see, for homeostasis to work, there has to be a feedback loop back to the brain to wind things up or down according to need. What happens with repeated episodes of stress or trauma is that the feedback loop doesn't work as well and the balance is switched more to up than down, more to on than off. Sometimes this is made worse because the imbalance induces an epigenetic change which makes the genes driving the adrenal gland increase production of more cortisol than the body needs. What you're left with is a chronically switched-on stress system, which can make us eat more, drink more alcohol, raise our blood pressure, and seriously stretch parts of the brain. The stretched bits are the ones which make memory work (the hippocampus), facilitate learning and emotion (amygdala), and allow us to plan and make sensible decisions (the prefrontal cortex).

The psychology of what some call 'allostatic load' has been described as 'anticipation'. The analogy here is getting out of bed. When we wake up in the morning and think about getting out of bed, our body anticipates this and adjusts our blood pressure control so we don't faint when we stand up after a night lying flat. If we've experienced a lot of stressful adversity, our brain and the rest of the body switch to a high level of anticipation that trouble is coming, which for many people is not an unrealistic proposition. The side effects are worry, fear and anxiety, and possibly even drug and alcohol use. It's like a broken thermostat and when we are challenged we don't respond as effectively as we might.

The result is wear and tear on our body including our brain – allostatic load – and it's a whole person picture of risk rather than dissecting things down to individual factors such as cholesterol, blood sugar and blood pressure. Allostatic load is hard to measure, but studies following the health and wellbeing of thousands of people in countries such as China, Taiwan, the US and Scotland have found increased rates of premature death associated with high allostatic load, and often the causes of death are wide ranging. The Scottish study even took deprivation into account and for every unit increase in allostatic load, the all-cause death rate went up by 8 per cent. Allostatic load was a stronger predictor of dying younger than you should, compared to most individual risk factors.

The good news

The good news is that allostatic load can be reversible, in part thanks to neuroplasticity – the ability of networks of nerves in the brain to change according to circumstance.

Exercise: There is evidence, for instance, that exercise can reverse some of the effects of allostatic load. MRI scans of the brain in action have shown that people's thinking ability improved as did their decision-making and planning. Their prefrontal cortex (which in high allostatic load loses neural networks) increased in volume and grey matter.

Social integration: This is about having strong social networks which are diverse and therefore resilient to change. It's about reducing isolation and increasing the social contacts you have on a day-by-day and weekly basis. It's about family, friends, sociable neighbourhoods and belonging to groups and organisations. The evidence is that the more socially integrated you are, the lower your allostatic load, the slower your thinking and memory decline, perhaps the healthier your immune system and the longer you live in good health. There's been a long debate about whether it's social integration that's keeping you young or whether you have to be young at heart to get out and about and be socially active. In other words, the chicken or egg question – and it's made more complex because socially active people are also more physically active. While there's no doubt that once chronic diseases such as heart failure or dementia have set in, being socially active becomes hard. However, when large numbers of people have been followed for many years, it does look as though staying in work and maintaining social contacts does keep you younger longer. Government policy is important here too because if you have poor town planning, where housing is distant from the other activities of daily life and you can't just walk round the corner to see people or mix with friends, social integration becomes much harder than it needs to be.

Learning: The longer you go on in education when you're young, in general the longer you live in good health. In part this has something to do with lower allostatic load because more education tends to give you more job and income security and more control over your destiny. It's also that your brain develops more complex and deeper neural networks which stand you in good stead when you're older and, remember, keeping your youth starts above the neck. When you have time to do it, learning a new, complex skill like a language or a musical instrument stretches and extends your brain. Most people wait until they're retired to do that but if you can do it when you're much younger, you'll be laying important foundations for the future.

What and how you eat and how you cook it: This brings together physical activity (growing your own food or walking to the shops daily for the freshest produce), cooking slowly to avoid premature ageing from high temperature chemical changes (advanced glycation end products – see The Long-Life Kitchen Chemistry Set), maintaining a highly diverse diet, and eating with friends and family (social contact). As research progresses in the next few years, it should become clearer the extent to which the microbiome can influence allostasis.

Brain vs brawn

#ormaybeboth

There is abundant evidence that being physically fit helps you to live younger and longer. A review of studies involving nearly 43,000 elite athletes in a variety of sports from team games to track and field to power events to Tour de France entrants – with a bias towards males in the samples, found a 27 per cent reduction in deaths from heart disease, 40 per cent reduction in the risk of cancer and a 33 per cent reduced risk of dying from any cause at a given age. This is similar to recreational athletes who have a 27 per cent reduced risk of premature death. There is also evidence of lower use of medications for chronic diseases. The data are complicated by the fact the athletes tend not to smoke or drink too much and eat a healthy diet, but most studies try to control for those effects and have concluded that fitness is a factor in its own right.

A fascinating Australian study wanted to see whether you lived longer if you were a *brain* athlete. They compared data on 15,000 Olympic medallists in physical sports with 1200 international chess grandmasters. The researchers also took into account where they came from, since grandmasters are traditionally Eastern Europeans – a particularly unhealthy part of the world. The findings were that, at age 30, chess grandmasters had a significantly longer life expectancy than the general population overall and certainly longer than people in their home region. Interestingly, at age 30, their life expectancy was no less than Olympic medallists. There is also evidence that grandmasters have less dementia, which shouldn't be a surprise since chess is a highly complex set of cognitive tasks.

Before you get too excited about these findings if your sport is chess, there are some caveats. Grandmasters are mostly men, which means you can't necessarily extrapolate to women, and they also do take care of themselves and often have a nutritionist and trainer looking after their physical wellbeing.

There are also 'psychological pay-offs', as well as greater wealth, but that might also fit well with the idea of keeping allostasis in balance.

Your move – and the timer is on …

Don't open up the BAG – mental health and living younger longer

#mindthegap

Quick take: The brain is no exception to the general rule that you can be biologically younger or older than your chronological age. Some researchers call this the brain age gap (BAG), usually measured by an MRI scan looking at how much connectivity you have between nerves and neural networks in the brain compared to what you'd expect for a person's age. A youthful brain has rich connections and deep networks allowing high performance thinking and memory. It's also associated with good mental health and wellbeing. Diabetes is associated with accelerated brain ageing and there's growing evidence that severe mental health issues may also increase the brain age gap. The BAG is not inevitable and is preventable.

The view depends on your vantage point: Nobel Laureate Dan Kahneman and his collaborator, the late Amos Tversky, who together researched the psychology of risk perception, found that human beings are naturally loss averse. We become disproportionately and sometimes irrationally more distressed by the idea that we might lose something like our health or money than the idea that we might actually gain health or wealth, nice though that thought might be. And so it is with getting older. When you're relatively young and fit and you look ahead to your future ageing self, what you imagine it might be like can feel more distressing than it actually will be. That's because all you see is loss of health and wellbeing, which is not as inevitable as you think. When older people look ahead, while they've probably got a few aches and pains and take pills for their cholesterol, they often realise what they have is not as bad as they anticipated. As people age they seem to become happier, which might seem like a paradox when you're 40.

Men and women who live long and healthy lives usually have young and healthy brains for their age and it shows in their mental health. Sardinians, who tend to have a longer than average life expectancy, at least in part because of their genes, have less cognitive decline than you'd expect, apart from not coping with change as well as they used to. They also have high levels of psychological and emotional wellbeing. Repeated studies of people who live to extreme old age show similar findings, namely that – along with being reasonably fit and having good thinking and memory for their age – they have high levels of psychological wellbeing. They feel quite happy and there's some evidence that – on average when you look at populations – the longer you live, the happier and more satisfied with life you tend to be.

Mental wellness and living longer: In most rich countries, mental health issues such as depression, self-harm and suicide are up there in the highest causes of lost years of life. That's because mental illness disproportionately affects younger people and when they die, more years of life are lost than when a 75-year-old has a heart attack. So finding ways to prevent psychological issues – through interventions in pregnancy and childhood, improving educational opportunities, strengthening communities to find ways of helping young people belong and support each other, as well as avoiding the early uptake of alcohol and other drugs – will extend life expectancy.

The effects of mental health issues on a healthy lifespan go far beyond self-harm and suicide, tragic and preventable as they are. For instance, people with severe mental health issues like schizophrenia have a high rate of chronic diseases like diabetes and heart disease because their physical health is not well cared for and their medications can have significant side effects. In fact, according to a review of the evidence, the life expectancy gap for people with schizophrenia is about 20 years compared to the rest of the population.

But back to the brain age gap. Because mental health issues do seem to affect it. When people with major depression have been studied, their brains seemed significantly older on scanning than their chronological age. Now that's not proof of cause and effect but the worse the depression, the bigger the BAG. That also goes along with shorter telomeres and epigenetic changes associated with oxidative stress – again very tangible physical correlations with psychological problems. Studies have found similar gaps linked to schizophrenia, post traumatic stress disorder (PTSD) and anxiety but interestingly not with bipolar disorder. In these studies, as people living with these conditions got older, there was also an increased risk of problems with thinking and memory. The brain age gap seems to take time to show itself and is more pronounced in older people than younger, which is good news for prevention and early treatment, assuming there is a cause and effect relationship. There's evidence that antidepressant medications can reduce the gap and improve cognitive performance in people with depression. There's also some evidence that psychotherapy can close the BAG and there's little doubt about the effects of exercise on the brain.

Feeling positive about optimism?

#wishfulthinking?

Optimists are generally people who expect good things to happen but there are a few myths about optimism. People often assume that a person's attitude of mind matters when, for example, they have cancer. This can put pressure on the person with cancer when they're made to feel bad if they're not feeling optimistic or positive all the time. Reassuringly, Australian research has shown that optimism makes no difference to cancer outcomes whereas being clinically depressed does. Why that's reassuring is that you can't force someone to be an optimist but you can treat depression.

With longevity it may be a different story. Long-term, large studies of tens of thousands of women and men, following them for up to 30 years, have found that the more optimistic you are, the longer you live. Comparing the most optimistic people to the least, there was a 15 per cent increase in lifespan and a 50–70 per cent better chance of surviving to age 85. This is not proof of cause and effect but the studies did try to take account of other lifestyle factors in an optimist's life. Why optimism might extend lifespan is not known but is probably increased uptake of anti-ageing factors such as physical activity, social engagement and other lifestyle influences, even though the studies did try to control for them. The thing is that you can't just dial up optimism. Sometimes you might need to work on the perceived negative stuff in your life before you can move to a more positive outlook. That's what cognitive behavioural therapy is particularly good at.

Goldilocks and sleep – what's 'just right' for living long?

#readthesmallprint

Quick nap: When you look at the scientific literature, there's evidence that habitual short sleep (fewer than five or six hours a night) and long sleep (nine hours or more) are associated with dying prematurely from several causes. What research suggested seemed to be going on with people who slept long was that they had a medical problem underlying the sleep issue and that could have been the real reason for the increased risk of premature death. Short sleep, on the other hand, couldn't be blamed on dementia or heart disease and was a problem in its own right. The Goldilocks spot for sleep, according to studies done a few years ago, is around seven hours a night of total sleep time. But before you get too excited, this sweet spot is not so much the sleep duration which makes you live longer, it's the length of sleep at which there's no *increased* risk of prematurely dying. Now ... you've got to be really careful about sleep research because there are lots of issues with it. For example, many studies rely on people self-reporting their sleep habits and that can be unreliable. Sleep studies are also notorious for extrapolating your destiny from a single measure of sleep at one particular point in time. Even the better studies only assess sleep twice a few years apart. More recent research, though, has dug further and found that there are other things going on in what people say is short and long sleep. For example, it turns out that many of the people who say they sleep more than nine hours a night are actually not sleeping for all that time. Sure, they're lying in bed for nine hours or more but are having trouble sleeping. Basically they have insomnia. People who say they sleep fewer than six hours are often actually experiencing poor sleep quality and that's probably the issue rather than duration. That's good news, in fact, since while sleep therapy is fairly good at improving sleep quality and insomnia, it's pretty crap at increasing the number of actual sleep hours a short sleeper gets.

It's not entirely clear why we sleep but the evidence points to the need for reprocessing, restoration, a chemical clean-up in the brain and rest. Human beings have, like most animals, their own timekeeping system adapted to the 24-hour day, known as 'circadian rhythm' (see Keeping Time). It's generated by a 'clock' in the brain which responds to light. Light from our eyes is turned into electrical signals in nerves which pass near the pineal gland, which produces the hormone melatonin when it's dark. Melatonin goes up at night before sleep and is one reason you want your bedroom to be really dark and free of screens, the light from which can confuse the pineal into thinking it's daytime.

In addition, we each have our own chronotype, the tendency to be a morning or evening person. When it comes to living younger longer, research suggests that being a morning person is better, which is tough news for evening people and night-owls because your chronotype is hard to change. There is evidence that night-owls have a higher risk of diabetes and heart disease, but a large British study of 433,000 adults aged from 38 to 73 and followed for over six years, looked specifically at the chances of dying prematurely. It took into account all sorts of factors like smoking, obesity, wealth, education and sleep duration, and found that when you compared the most evening-type people with the most morning-type people (i.e. the furthest ends of the scale), night-owls had more chronic illnesses and psychological issues and about a 10 per cent increased risk of dying from any cause. There's a reasonable influence of genes on chronotype but the explanation probably has more to do with diet, exercise and work. Night-owls tend to peak in the late afternoon to early evening and have a habit of skipping breakfast. They also don't eat as much fruit and vegetables. A delay in mealtimes, particularly dinner, might also add to your circadian misalignment because if you eat late it can make it harder to go to sleep. Eating a big meal close to our natural 'rest phase' can throw out our internal rhythms and can be linked to obesity and other metabolic problems. There might also be behavioural patterning if you grew up in a household of late bedders. Chronotype is not immutable, which is good news for parents of adolescents who are still gaming at 1 a.m.

I tell you this because when you start to talk about sleep and living longer, it gets murky and chronotype is just one of the factors which makes it more complicated.

There's also an association between sleep and an increased risk of dementia. For example, a study of 5000 MRI brain scans in 1300 healthy people with normal thinking and memory, who had repeat scans anywhere between three and 11 years apart, found a link between poor sleep quality, daytime tiredness and wasting (atrophy) of the hippocampus, which is an essential part of the brain involved in cognitive function. Doesn't mean the poor sleep quality caused the dementia but there is something going on. There's also evidence that fewer than six hours sleep a night is associated with dementia and the build-up of tau and beta amyloid, the two substances that accumulate in the brains of people with Alzheimer's disease. Again, you can't jump to the assumption that this is cause and effect. The subtle signs of dementia can start earlier in life and dementia itself affects sleep cycles. So short sleep may be the result not the cause of the dementing process.

Your age, work, health and fitness, whether you have young kids, and your gender (men sleep less than women) all affect how much sleep you have and whether it's good quality. Disrupted sleep patterns are common in people with depression and anxiety. Anxiety can prevent you from falling asleep in the first place, while waking up in the middle of the night and ruminating on negative thoughts may be a sign of depression.

So let's try to zero in on sleep itself.

Extensive reviews have brought together the available evidence on sleep and mortality, following large numbers of people across a range of countries for many years and recording lots of variables in their lifestyles. Until recently these reviews largely found the same thing, namely that short sleepers (usually defined as fewer than five or six hours a night) and long sleepers (usually defined as nine or more hours per night) had increased chances of dying – short sleepers by 12 per cent and long sleepers by up to 30 per cent. The data on short sleep seemed to show that it was not so much caused by factors like illness. It looked more like the lack of sleep itself was the problem causing the premature ageing, perhaps triggering inflammation and oxidative stress. There are also animal studies showing that with severe sleep loss, the gut microbiome shifts to bacteria which are more likely to throw off reactive oxygen species – the substances that cause oxidative stress.

The data on long sleepers, on the other hand, did suggest that the issue was caused by ill health. They were older and sicker, more depressed and fatigued, got less exercise, and were more likely to have obstructive sleep apnoea. So it was assumed that in long sleepers the physical and psychological problems were the core reasons for dying sooner. The startling and hardly comforting conclusion of one review was that six to eight hours sleep per night is not associated with harm! Now there's a resounding recommendation. If you, like me, are a six-hour or less sleeper, before you go into a cold panic and update your will, here's an idea of how messy this research is.

The individual studies they brought together varied a lot in their findings. Sleep was self-reported, which is not ideal as you'll find out below. Sleep also tended only to be measured once during studies that may have lasted for decades.

Is it sleep or sleep difficulties which are the problem? A recent study of more than a million people in the US, UK and the Netherlands tried to iron out some of these research issues and get to the heart of what might be going on by more accurately measuring stuff around sleep as well as sleep itself. Unlike other studies, they did not find a huge epidemic of sleep deprivation. Only 6 per cent of people slept outside what they reckoned was an acceptable range of six to 11 hours a night. If you looked at the recommended range, which is more like seven to eight hours a night, then 25 per cent of the people slept less than that; while this is a lot, it isn't the almost 50 per cent whoppingly suggested by other studies. The researchers also confirmed what sleep therapists have known for some time, which is that sleep quality and duration are more influenced by the time you go to bed than the time you get up. Waketimes don't change that much during life while bedtimes do, which is why sleep therapy tends to focus on what time you got to bed the night before.

Anyway, when they looked more closely at what was being called short and long sleep, it turned out that there was more than sleep happening for those people. So-called short sleepers complained of feeling they had poor sleep quality, which is hard to define because it's a perceived thing but generally means feeling unrefreshed and tired in the morning and maybe having an interrupted night's sleep. Jobs, mental health issues, traffic noise, drug and alcohol intake and poor sleep hygiene can all play a role.

So-called long sleepers often turned out not to be long sleepers at all, even though they were spending nine or more hours a night in bed. They were tossing and turning and complained of insomnia, which is defined by trouble falling asleep or trouble staying asleep that's been going on at least three nights a week for at least three months and interferes with your ability to function normally during the day, leaving you feeling irritable or unable to concentrate. Insomnia can be due to factors such as changed life circumstances, loss, traumatic events, side effects of a variety of prescribed medications, general medical conditions, and mental health issues such as anxiety or depression.

While other studies have hinted that sleep quality and difficulties may be at least as important as sleep duration, their link to living younger longer is unproven. What's fascinating, though, is that the best sleep therapy often doesn't actually change your sleep duration. It gives you a better night's sleep.

The core elements of sleep therapy are cognitive behavioural therapy designed for insomnia (CBT-I), stimulus control therapy, sleep hygiene and sleep restriction.

Changing your thinking: Just like the CBT used for other problems like depression, CBT-I is about changing thoughts which are counterproductive to a good night's sleep. It helps people stop catastrophising in the middle of the night about their lack of sleep.

Bedrooms are for beds: Stimulus control therapy is pairing the bed with sleep, so only go to bed when you're tired, don't use it as the venue to work, watch a movie, to read on your iPad or chat on the phone.

Less sleep may be more: Sleep restriction therapy is a strict method of setting a fixed wake-up time in the morning and finding a time to go to bed when you're tired enough that you sleep right through to that set waketime. An unbroken sleep feels more refreshing and is probably more important than the number of hours of sleep. We all have a biological sleep drive that builds up and grows before we go to bed and if we stick to the routine, it stabilises our internal body clock. Research suggests that stimulus control and sleep restriction combined are the most powerful components of getting people to sleep better. If you're trying sleep restriction, you might need some guidance, as it requires discipline.

Tidy things up: Sleep hygiene is about leaving your phone or tablet in the living room, or in a place you can't hear or see it, making your bedroom dark, not working in bed and avoiding television when you can't sleep. It also involves reducing stimulants close to bedtime, like coffee and alcohol (that glass of wine or three might be keeping you awake or could be waking you up early), and not taking exercise too close to bedtime.

Say no to sleeping pills (mostly): Drugs are rarely the way to treat sleep quality and insomnia. They don't give you a normal night's sleep, have side effects and some can cause dependence. Sleep therapy works better and is longer lasting. Sometimes a sleeping pill can break the cycle but that's really all.

And the results are: Fixing your sleep may or may not make you live longer, but you'll certainly live a lot better. This still begs the question about your body clock – your circadian rhythm – which does much more to your body than get you off to sleep. It may be one of the things controlling how fast you age.

Keeping time – your body clocks and staying young

#timingmaybeeverything
#dontletnightbecomeday

In a tick: There are clocks pretty much everywhere in the body and there's a growing amount of research suggesting they play a key role in how quickly or slowly you age. Body clocks put your temperature up and down during the day and, among many other things, vary your iron levels, how sticky your blood is, how active and 'inflamed' your immune system is, and maybe even the function of cells in your joints, increasing or decreasing your risk of arthritis. These clocks affect the chemistry of ageing I described earlier in the sections on anti-ageing substances and dietary restriction. Clocks increase or decrease the speed at which cells age and whether they go into damaging hibernation (see Putting Out the Garbage). The master clock is in the brain and responds to light in our environment. Remembering that the mind and body are 'one' – a single entity – you won't be surprised to hear that the master clock (called the suprachiasmatic nucleus or SCN) then sends messages to the rest of the body through hormones in the blood, and at higher speed via our nerves – our electrical cabling. Getting your clock – your circadian rhythm – in order may be an important part of staying young. It would be sobering if middle-of-the-night screen time, our never-dark environment and street light streaming into your bedroom through inadequate window blinds were to age you prematurely. A healthy body clock is more than getting a good night's sleep. It's also about what and when we eat, how and when we exercise, and the interaction of the body clock with our psychological wellbeing, including whether we're chronically stressed.

There's a rhythm to life. The rhythm we're aware of operates at the level of mealtimes, days and nights, summer/winter, learning, work and rest, family dynamics and so on. There are rhythms, though, that happen below the level of our consciousness and operate at both high and medium speeds in almost every tissue of the body and they're often affected by these conscious, more obvious rhythms of life.

You've got to think about your body clock and be conscious of it because modern life fights against it. Street lighting, scarcity of dark environments, screen time late at night, eating patterns (e.g. restricted eating and loading everything into dinner) and exercising too late at night all may give your brain the wrong timing signals. Add chronic stress and you have a serious recipe for screwing up your clock.

The master clock – the SCN – is in your brain and responds to light. It sits just above where the nerves taking light from your eyes cross over on their way to the back of the brain to be processed into images. The clock evolved to respond to day/ night cycles – light and darkness – and literally keeps an eye on these cycles on behalf of the rest of the body. These cycles are called your circadian rhythm.

We tend to think about this master clock in terms of sleep, jet lag when we travel overseas and what's called our chronotype, which, crudely, is about whether you're a morning person or an evening one. But it's much more than that. When you eat and what you eat make a difference, and in almost every part of the body there are clock genes which march to their own drum beat as well as the rhythm coming from the brain. Protein synthesis, chronic stress hormones (cortisol in particular), fat and energy metabolism, cell proliferation and cancer control, blood pressure and the molecular processes of ageing, including inflammation, are all under the influence of our body clocks. In animal experiments, restricted feeding can shift the body clock, as can a high fat diet. Mental health is also affected and it goes beyond seasonal affective disorder where people become depressed during winter. General depression and bipolar disorder are also related to abnormalities in circadian rhythm.

Ageing itself has an effect on circadian rhythm which is thought to be due to oxidative stress and inflammation damaging the SCN – the master clock. The tendency is for us to shift from being evening people when we're young, to becoming morning people with a corresponding change to increased alertness in the early hours of the day. This may not be inevitable and there is some evidence that people who are ageing healthily experience less of that rhythm shift. Dementia and Alzheimer's disease are notorious for being associated with switched day/night cycles and it may be that disturbances in circadian rhythms increase the risk of dementia in the first place.

So … what does this mean practically?

Well, we need to shield ourselves from an environment which works against our body clocks. Having a darkened room with heavy curtains is not just about a better sleep. It's about forcing a better rhythm.

Screens at night take on an added toxicity as they mess with our day/night cycle.

Maintaining the best health we can, with the lowest levels of inflammation, from our early years on may slow the ageing of our body clocks and that's through exercise, possibly best in daylight, thinking about our mealtimes, eating a largely plant-based diet cooked with ingredients that enhance its anti-inflammatory effects, trying to restrict calories, and being careful with fasting and time-restricted eating.

In terms of therapy for issues such as non-seasonal depression and dementia, it may be possible to shift circadian rhythm with timed exposure to light and attention to eating times, but it's too early to know how much change is possible once ageing rhythms have set in. The use of melatonin – the brain hormone produced in response to darkness – as an anti-ageing medication is controversial and unproven.

Keeping your brain young

#alzheimersatbay
#notrocketscience
#sudokudoesntcutit

Remember, the mind and body are one. So what happens below your neck affects your brain and vice versa. For years the experts have said that a healthy heart equals a healthy brain and they've been right. As heart disease has declined in many countries so has the incidence of dementia. Doesn't prove cause and effect but it is one of the factors. Studies of brain scans comparing chronological age with the state of the brain and dementia have shown that diabetes, heart disease, high blood pressure and depression all increase the risk of accelerated brain ageing, and physical strength is protective probably because it's a marker of a healthy lifestyle.

While specific studies of diet and brain ageing are hard to pin down, there is evidence that a Mediterranean dietary pattern high in natural antioxidants and B vitamins and low in salt is associated with slower brain ageing.

Exercising your whole brain by learning new complex skills like a language or musical instrument does help develop brain resilience by expanding neural networks. Narrow tasks like sudoku puzzles probably don't exercise enough of your brain to make a difference. While your genes do play a role in how well your brain ages, recent research suggests that the more education you've had, the lower the effects of 'bad' genes. And if you're a parent, the longer you can keep your kids in education the better for their long-term brain health.

Metabolic stress from intense exercise also appears to be associated with a younger brain. It's less clear that intermittent fasting is as good for your brain as often touted. While it may work in animals, it's far from clear in humans. On the other hand, calorie restriction without compromising your nutrition may be of benefit.

Alcohol is pretty poisonous for the brain and gets more so as you age and have lower reserves to deal with a heavy night on the turps. Not smoking goes without saying, and keeping your blood pressure down through exercise, being careful about weight and your salt intake and if necessary through medication all make a big difference to risk.

There are many brain training programs on the market and some have been shown to improve cognitive abilities or to slow decline. The better ones help you with lifestyle changes including sleep, and it may be that the sleep component is more potent than the brain training itself. But be wary, the quality of studies into brain training is generally low and a recent review of the evidence found that the effects were modest.

PART 9

Here's what you can do at any age

#duuuhh

Short answer: Do every preventive thing you can. Hard to live younger longer if you die of a preventable disease first. No point in cooking up a Mediterranean storm or doing F45 classes if you're going to die young from, say, a preventable cancer. What follows below assumes you're doing the basics around dietary pattern, cuisine, regular frugality and reasonably intense exercise. Be careful in the sun as it may age more than your skin. Look up the current advice for the amount of sun exposure needed to maintain your vitamin D levels.

Here's what you can do in your 20s

Now's the best time to do stuff that will help you live younger longer.

* Don't smoke burnt plants of any kind or vape crap that was never meant to be burnt. Try not to use alcohol or other drugs to the extent that they change your mental state. Getting drunk or high are signs of binge use, which is not good for your brain health.
* Get as much formal education as you can. It reduces your chances of dementia when you're older or, at the least, delays it and can possibly counteract the effect of genes you might have inherited which increase the risk of dementia.
* At least once in your 20s, get your GP to check your blood pressure and cholesterol in case you need to change your eating, alcohol intake and exercise levels.
* Start the habit of eating a plant-based diet with not too much red meat. Now's the time to get into the habit of mild calorie restriction in association with moderately intense exercise. The easy way might be intermittent frugality every three days or so (see Intermittent Frugality). Also a plant-based diet is in itself low in calories relative to the nutrition you get and satisfying.
* Exercise for 45 minutes to an hour most days of the week, reasonably intensively, and include muscle

strengthening in each session. Now's the time to get into the habit of developing and maintaining strong muscles.

* Watch your weight (see calorie restriction above).
* Avoid food fads and be careful about time-restricted eating which, along with screen time, may screw up your body clocks and start an accelerated ageing process.
* Severely limit screen use after dark, make sure your bedroom doesn't let in street lighting and don't mess with mealtimes. In other words, get your circadian rhythm into shape. It's good for both mental and physical health.
* Seek help for depression and anxiety if you're experiencing them. Depression, in particular, may contribute to accelerated ageing.
* In your 20s, your elderly relatives are likely to still be alive. Now's the time to find out who in your family died of what and at what age, so you can get an idea of any genetic risk you could have inherited. Seek genetic counselling if something does turn up.
* Don't assume that because you're young, you're not at risk of anything. Any lumps, bleeding, bruising, unexplained weight loss or pain, see your GP.
* Start cervical cancer screening when you're 25, assuming you've been sexually active.
* Get yourself a good GP whom you trust and like.

Here's what you can do if you're a parent or plan to become one

Most of the above plus ...

* Stop smoking if you've started. The first ten cigarettes are the most harmful so you've got to quit altogether. Avoid alcohol and other drugs if you're trying to have a baby and minimise them afterwards.
* Make sure your blood pressure and weight are normal.
* Eat a Mediterranean-style diet.
* Exercise at moderate intensity, including strength training, for 45 minutes most days of the week.
* Women of childbearing age should be taking folate supplements.
* Avoid maternal obesity. It's associated with accelerated ageing in the offspring, with increased risks of diabetes and premature death from heart disease.
* Take actions which will optimise the birth weight of your baby so that he or she will have healthy organs which will stand them in good stead for the rest of their lives. That includes having a normal blood pressure, not putting on too much weight during pregnancy, and not smoking or drinking any alcohol during pregnancy.
* Encourage your kids to get as much education as possible so they enter adulthood with healthy brains which have deep resilience.

* If you have a healthy diet, that's what your kids should eat too.
* Encourage good sleep patterns in your kids and no late night screen time.
* If you haven't got a good GP you like and trust, try hard to find one.

Here's what you can do in your 30s and 40s

* Don't smoke burnt plants (do I really need to explain why again?).
* If you've got kids, encourage them to continue in education as long as they can. The more you're educated, the longer you live and the later you develop dementia.
* If you've got kids, make sure they're fully immunised, including to hepatitis B and human papillomavirus (HPV), both of which are anti-cancer vaccines.
* Find a GP you like and stick with them. You need someone who knows you and cares about your health with a laser focus.
* Women should continue in cervical cancer screening. No bottle of supplements is going to match screening to prevent you dying prematurely of an avoidable cancer.
* Know what your cholesterol levels are – the good (HDL) and the bad (LDL). A high LDL in your 30s can indicate you're already silting up your arteries

and need to lose weight (lowers unhealthy fats), change your diet and up the exercise (raises HDL). If your cholesterol is really high, you may have a genetic problem and need medication.

* Know what your blood pressure is. There's nothing like a constant battering from high blood pressure to age your brain, heart and kidneys prematurely and leave you open to life-shortening heart attacks, strokes and dementia. If your blood pressure is getting beyond normal levels, then lose weight (can have the equivalent effect of a blood pressure med), exercise for 45 minutes to an hour of moderate intensity most days of the week (also reduces blood pressure), lower your alcohol intake or switch to low alcohol drinks, and reduce your salt intake.

* Don't sit on symptoms like bleeding, bruising, unplanned loss of weight or new onset of pain just because you're young.

Here's what you can do if you're 50

* All of the above, plus breast and bowel cancer screening.
* Keep eating a very diverse diet … Don't allow it to become narrowed down because you can't be bothered. That's what tends to happen as you get older.
* Same goes for exercise. You're now entering the time of life when your muscles – if you don't work on them – get weaker and smaller. If anything, you

should be upping the amount and intensity (carefully tuned to your capacity and level of fitness).

* Keep your abdominal fat as low as possible as measured by your waist circumference (see Your Abdomen and Staying Young).

* Look around you and assess how many people you can call upon if you need help or support. Now's the time to maintain and work on family and friendships rather than take them for granted. Social interaction and support are central to staying young.

* At age 50 there are five factors which predict a longer life in health:
– a BMI between 18.5 and 24.9
– 30 minutes or more per day of moderate to vigorous exercise
– alcohol intake in line with official recommendations
– a high quality diet (e.g. Mediterranean)
– never smoked

* Women who have none of these factors live just over 23 years more free of diabetes, heart disease or cancer; men get 23.5 years. Women who have four or five of these factors live 34 years free of these diseases; for men, it's 31 years extra.

Here's what you can do if you're 60, 70 – or indeed 80 or 90

* Do all of the above, especially increasing the focus on a diverse diet and exercise with lots of muscle

strengthening. Strong muscles are critical for slowing down the path to frailty and maybe even avoiding it altogether. Really focus on a varied, Mediterranean dietary pattern.

* Most cancer screening programs stop in your 70s. That's because the clinical trials didn't include people over 70. It doesn't mean that cancer screening stops being useful. It may even have better pay-offs for individuals since cancer becomes more common as you age. You don't want unnecessarily intrusive treatment for a cancer that's been diagnosed late when it could have been found early. Public health people talk about populations and years of life gained for the investment in a screening program. Obviously, there are large numbers of years to be gained when a 50-year-old is diagnosed rather than a 75-year-old. But that doesn't take account of the benefits for an individual, assuming the treatment isn't more risky than the cancer. Take your GP's advice on this but let me tell you, I'm not stopping cancer screening.

* Immunisations such as pneumococcal and shingles are also important.

* Learning a new and complex skill like playing a musical instrument or a language deepens the neural networks in your brain.

* Focus on your circadian rhythm and getting a consolidated night's sleep, even if it's not as long as you'd like.

* Work on ways to broaden your group of friends. Social networks are an important part of staying young.

The annual check-up and staying young ...

#mostlybullshit

Quick one: There seems to be this idea that you should see your doctor each year for a check-up and some companies spend a fortune on this. With a few exceptions – mainly to do with monitoring you if you have a chronic illness like diabetes, heart disease or cancer – there's little, if any, evidence that the annual check-up makes any difference and there's actually potential for harm.

One problem with the annual check-up when you're healthy is that they can't even get the name straight. There are a variety of terms used: check-up, health check, periodic health examinations, wellness visits, annual physicals and routine visits, to mention a few. In addition, there's little standardisation about what happens in one of these visits. Some corporate checks leave no flap of skin or orifice unexamined and draw blood for a swathe of tests and some even will do a cardiac stress test, a CT scan of the heart and occasionally even a whole-body MRI. The more tests, the more impressed some people are when, in fact, their reaction should be the opposite. Many tests in well people are more likely to detect a meaningless abnormality which leads to more tests and procedures with more risk of harm, the further down the radiology and pathology road you go. In the United States, an astounding one in ten doctor visits are for a routine check-up.

A recent review of the international evidence from randomised trials and observing groups of people looked at whether there were tangible benefits from the annual check-up or regular review in an otherwise well person. The studies involved many thousands of people with a follow-up from six months to 30 years. What was done at these visits varied a lot and included blood and urine screens, eye checks, physical examinations and sometimes even meeting with a behaviour coach.

The vast majority of studies showed no reduction in premature deaths, although there was increased detection of chronic diseases such as high blood pressure, diabetes, depression and chronic kidney disease. Detection didn't necessarily mean the chronic diseases were well treated. In the years that followed, there were very small differences in weight, cholesterol and blood pressure. However, two trials of older people did show a small mortality benefit, but don't get too excited. In a four-year follow-up the difference in risk was between 1 and 3 per cent.

On the other side of the ledger, annual check-ups are not necessarily harm-free.

A Danish study of 59,000 people found a higher rate of premature death in women but there was no obvious reason. Another study found increased stroke rates. It could be that sicker people go for check-ups, but they tried to allow for that. The problem is that if too many uncalled-for tests are done, you risk finding something that looks worrying but in fact isn't. However, chasing that down could require lots more tests which themselves can take you on wild goose chases and worry. Occasionally, this can even result in needless surgery.

That doesn't mean getting to know your GP and them getting to know you isn't a good idea. It is. It's also a good idea every few years (no-one really knows the right number) to check in with them to make sure that you're not putting on too much weight around your waist, and your blood pressure and your blood fats (cholesterol and triglycerides) are okay. The proviso is that this all changes if you have a strong family history of a particular disease or have had a problem in the past and need surveillance. Obviously, any new symptom that you're worried about needs to be seen asap but that's very different from routine check-ups every year when you're otherwise well.

Keep your bullshit meter on high alert

#saveyourmoney

Okay, you're expecting me to dump the proverbial on a whole heap of stuff from colonic irrigation to detoxifying yourself, to shutting yourself in a tepee while someone rings gongs, to ayahuasca-fuelled weekends spent hallucinating and vomiting.

Well, I'm not going to. Just stay sensible and sceptical. Unless you're in kidney or liver failure, your body is pretty good at detoxification. There might be something to psychedelics for depression but they're unlikely to affect healthy brain ageing one way or other. Group activities are good for making new friends and contacts. If you've got this far in the book, you'll realise that at the moment it's not worth shelling out for anti-ageing supplements. You could inadvertently take them in ways that speed rather than slow ageing.

Spend the money you've saved on a Mediterranean cookbook and guitar lessons to expand your brain. Harder work than swallowing a pill but far more likely to have an effect.

PART 10

The air we breathe

#forgetthisatourperil
#thewindsknownoborders

The dirt on dirt: Air pollution causes – on average – nearly three years of life lost per person around the world. Some of that is hard to prevent, such as from bushfires and volcanoes, but stopping human-made air pollution, which is largely due to the burning of fossil fuels, would reduce that loss by more than half. The impact of air pollution is up there with tobacco and much more than that of violence.

Pollution from all sources (including tainted water, work exposure and heavy metal contamination) caused 9 million premature deaths globally in 2015. That was 16 per cent of total global deaths that year – and three times more deaths than AIDs, tuberculosis and malaria together; 15 times as many deaths as war and violence; more than twice as many early deaths as caused by a high salt diet and similarly for obesity. The only traditional health factors which were more deadly than pollution were all dietary risk factors together and high blood pressure. It equates to 254 million years of life lost and 14 million years lost to disability. To put that into personal terms, on days of high air pollution the increased risk of dying prematurely on that day and the five days following may be around 3 per cent. Doesn't sound much until I remind you that's over just a few days. About 170,000 people die each year in Australia. Let's say that's 460 a day. A high day of air pollution could mean 13 or 14 more people die than otherwise would have on that day and that doesn't take account of the children and young people suffering damage which could shorten their lives in the long run. In the years since 2015, many experts in the field feel it has only become worse.

Eliminating fossil fuel burning would solve a lot of this. While the majority of these deaths are in low to middle income countries, many are still in wealthy nations. Laws and tough regulations are what have made the difference in high income countries and when a politician claims environmental rules need to be relaxed for economic development and jobs, they are not telling the truth, corrupt, ignorant of the economics of clean development, or a combination of the three. We in rich countries are under constant political risk of being thrust back into unsafe environments and dying younger rather than living longer. We run the risk of being beguiled into a false sense of security and forget that when public health and preventive measures like environmental regulation work, nothing happens. The trouble is that we only sit up when bad things happen and at that point deeply regret not having noticed or rejoiced in their absence.

Pollution and all that crap

Pollution is the accumulation of harmful substances in the environment. In a bygone world with few humans and no industry, pollution was largely airborne and came from natural events like volcanoes erupting. As humans stopped being hunter-gatherers and settled as farmers in growing towns and villages, human and animal poo became a major and smelly pollutant – although not fully recognised as dangerous until the 19th century. In fact, functioning toilets and waste management are still rarities in too many parts of the world. In Britain, it took a cholera epidemic in the 19th century and the evidence from a London doctor, John Snow (no, not Jon Snow for *Thrones* fans), in 1854 that it was caused by human waste contaminating the drinking water supply, to spur the development of a modern sewage system. As an aside, to illustrate the short lifespans in the 1800s, Snow died just four years later at the age of 45.

Settlement and the need to cook food and warm the household created intense and damaging indoor air pollution, which is still all too prevalent today in low income countries. Household air pollution from inefficient and poorly vented wood or dung stoves has been a significant cause of childhood deaths from pneumonia and adult deaths from lung and heart disease for thousands of years. Globally, indoor air pollution is still a major cause of premature death, not to mention the deforestation and environmental damage that goes with it.

The Industrial Revolution took pollution to a new level. Industry was fuelled by mining and ignored its polluting emissions and run-off. The revolution needed lead and other heavy metals. The smelting of lead and its widespread use reduced the IQ of generations of children. It also needed to burn coal on a massive scale to power the factories, and relied on the use of dangerous chemicals to process the iron and textiles. Chemical contamination of soil and the water supply alongside environmental air pollution became additional causes of premature deaths and still are in large swathes of the world. If you think that's an issue just for low and middle income countries, you'd be wrong. Since 1950 it's been estimated that 140,000 new chemicals have been introduced into the environment via industry and agriculture, with fewer than half having been tested for toxicity. The invention and adoption of the internal combustion engine to power trucks and cars added to the poisons in the air. Fossil fuel combustion produces fine particles which travel down to the smallest airways in the lungs and are absorbed into our bloodstreams, causing premature ageing, heart attacks, strokes, cancer and probably developmental issues in children.

The current debate about mitigating climate change and the supposed damage it will do to economic development is a convenient fallacy that's far from new. For a long time economists and politicians have argued, firstly, that environmental damage is an inevitable consequence of industrial development and, secondly, that regulating pollution will slow economic growth. Such pollution, in fact, reduces GDP and is a burden on health spending to the tune of \$240–600 billion per year globally. Repeated studies have shown that regulating pollution boosts economic growth rather than impedes it. For every dollar spent on mitigating air pollution, it's estimated that \$30 is saved. Taking lead out of the environment, for instance, has been estimated to have increased the IQ of children by 1–5 points with flow-on effects worth hundreds of billions of dollars in addition to the human benefits. Asbestos is another example of a potent carcinogen which, despite having been banned in some countries, is still used in exported building materials manufactured in some low to middle income nations.

There is no market for clean air, water or soils. Yes, in heavily polluted nations, rich people can live in safe enclaves and buy bottled water. In China, wealthy parents buy overseas milk formula for their babies. That, however, doesn't help the population at large and no-one can stop the wind. On some days, prevailing winds can carry coal pollution from China to California to the extent that 11 per cent of the western United States' black carbon pollution is imported. On magical Lake Como in Italy, there are fewer and fewer days when the air is clear. When there's market failure like this, the role of governments is to step in and pass laws and implement tough regulations to force industry to reduce the damage pollution does to the environment. That's what rich nations have done, although incompletely when it comes to fossil fuels and new chemicals. It's also fragile, as Americans discovered during the Trump presidency when the administration tried to circumvent or set aside environmental regulations in the name of industrial development and employment.

Fresh air

Repeated studies show a strong relationship between air pollution and dying prematurely and causing problems in children. An opportunistic experiment occurred in Utah where a steel mill closed and reopened and they were able to measure particulates in the air as they decreased and increased. When the particulate levels reached a certain point, hospital admissions for children tripled and doubled for adults, especially for respiratory conditions like pneumonia, pleurisy and asthma. Another study of six cities, which took into account smoking, found a 26 per cent increase in premature deaths in the most polluted city compared to the least, and that was from lung cancer, heart disease and chronic obstructive pulmonary disease.

The particles which cause the most concern are the tiniest ones – PM$_{2.5}$, which means they're 2.5 microns across. That's so small they get absorbed into the bloodstream from the lungs, induce oxidative stress (i.e. premature ageing), damage the lining of arteries, increase the risk of blood clots and, along with inhaling sulphur and nitrogen dioxide, are causally linked to raised heart disease rates. One study found that for every 10 micrograms of fine particulates per cubic metre, respiratory and heart disease mortality go up by 6 per cent and there's a direct correlation with traffic density. Household income and education levels are also related, probably both in their own right and because affordable housing when you're poor is often in polluted suburbs. There is also evidence that the risk from fine particles isn't exactly linear and the risk curve might be steeper at lower levels.

Cigarettes behave in this way. The most dangerous cigarettes are the first ten a day.

Of the 9 million premature deaths due to pollution in 2015 – equating to 254 million years of life lost – 6.5 million of those deaths were due to air pollution of all kinds and 4.2 million of those were due to fine particulates. These data come from the Global Burden of Disease Study. The estimates of the World Health Organization (WHO) are even higher. The only global risks higher than fine particle air pollution are combined dietary risk factors and high blood pressure. Be under no illusion, this air pollution arises from the burning of fossil fuels and, if nothing changes, premature deaths will continue to rise. While the highest rates are in low income countries, 3 million of these air pollution deaths each year occur in upper-middle to high income nations. And as I said, it spreads, since winds know no borders.

These deaths are mostly in people over 60 because the effects take a few years to kick in, although there is a spike in the 0–4 year age group and there are growing concerns that children's physical and intellectual development can be affected.

The International Agency for Research on Cancer, which grades the cancer-causing potential of chemicals, classifies ambient air pollution and fine particulates as Grade 1 carcinogens.

And there's more

There is still work to be done even in rich countries. Lead is still used, for instance, in car batteries and mobile phones. Mercury is another heavy metal that's common in the environment and contaminated sites are an ongoing issue. Pesticides and herbicides have not necessarily been well studied for their long-term toxicity and some persist for long periods in the environment. A recently noticed added concern with unknown effects is excreted pharmaceutical drugs in the environment.

Since there's a limit to what you and I can do about this as individuals, the Lancet Commission on Pollution and Health made several recommendations, including: setting targets for pollution prevention; focusing globally when giving funding and technical support to low income countries to make control a priority; better ways of monitoring pollution; and including pollution control in strategies for the prevention of heart disease, cancer, dementia and even diabetes. And they also call for the 'circular economy':

> The three core principles of the circular economy are preservation of natural capital by reducing use of non-renewable resources and ecosystem management; optimisation of resource yields by circulating products and materials so that they are shared and their lifecycles extended; and fostering system effectiveness by designing out pollution, greenhouse gas emissions, and toxic materials that damage health.
> *Lancet Commission on Pollution and Health (2018)*

Which, of course, leads us to climate change.

End note: Climate change, environmental stress, the abuse of medicine and living shorter

#actnow
#focusonwhatmatters

All of the above plus: Most of this book has been about stuff that while important and does make a difference to how long and youthfully we live, is not existential the way climate and environmental change and the abuses of modern medicine are. Every natural cycle on earth and which keeps us alive is under stress, from water to air to carbon to phosphorus and nitrogen. There are too many people for the planet to sustain. Overpopulation and the need to feed the world has created high throughput agriculture where, for example, chickens, pigs and humans mix intensively and exchange viruses fast and furiously with each other and animals in the wild. We are cutting down ancient forests to extend agricultural land which often claps out within a few years but in the meantime exposes humans to new animals and viruses. We do not control the trade in wild animals which can spread new diseases. We are living in a world which is now designed for regular pandemics. COVID-19 will have set back average life expectancy globally by one or two years. Future pandemics caused by new organisms from animals will do the same again and again. Our food supply is at risk from drought, floods, fires, temperature change, landslides, sea level rise and ocean warming. Sea rises will cause massive human migration and the potential for even more environmental disruption and exposure to new micro-organisms. Extreme heat will kill people and limit the ability of outdoor workers to do their jobs. If the natural cycles of water, carbon, phosphorus and nitrogen collapse, so will the future of many on our planet because agriculture will collapse as well. There will be more wars over resources with escalating risk that biowarfare germs and nuclear arms will be used. Technologies like CRISPR which allow cheap gene editing are putting biosecurity at risk. The nightmare scenario is a member of ISIS with a masters in biology and a few hundred thousand dollars for a low-end lab creating a mutant version of smallpox. Climate change will expand the geographic range of diseases like dengue and malaria and it's probably already happened with Japanese encephalitis. The abuse of medical technologies such as antibiotics could return us to a pre-antibiotic world which will make pandemics look like a little blip on life expectancy. The growth of expensive medical treatments which save lives at the expense of our immune systems creates a growing population who are vulnerable to new infections and an epidemiological springboard for their spread.

I can't tell you how sick I am of hearing that the above is needless panic, despite it being mainstream among researchers. Critics often justify their attacks by claiming that past predictions made about the environment and overpopulation didn't happen.

Human ingenuity and the market will get us through, they say, whether it be in food production or carbon storage. What these critics don't realise, in devaluing past predictions by saying they didn't come to pass, is that when preventive strategies work, nothing happens. Immunisation and maternal and child health strategies and economic development have reduced the speed of population growth by reducing the need for large families. Agriculture has become more efficient in parts of the world, although it hasn't stopped deforestation. Prevention and intervention have worked but it's not been enough. There's also a tacit assumption that the highest burden of this environmental stress will be carried by people in low to middle income countries who are already food insecure and living in highly degraded environments. If the pandemic has taught us anything, it's that crises are pretty lousy at recognising borders. We're in this together and we'll all be touched.

Most of the solutions require political will more than technological innovation. Fossil fuel burning – the cause of climate change – causes millions of years of lost life each year, equating to 4.2 million people dying prematurely every year – at least. Those are lives which could be saved, disabilities prevented and climate change mitigated all at the same time by rapidly moving to renewable energy sources. We'll live younger longer on a planet that will see less catastrophic change.

Poverty alleviation, sustainable agriculture, economic development and access to high value primary healthcare will continue to reduce family size, improve health and damage the environment less. If that's tied to high quality education, then that will even further enhance the reductions in poverty and improvements in health, wellbeing and longevity.

Multilateral cooperation and environmental surveillance could detect pandemic viruses when they first appear and reduce the chances of spread. Maybe the trust engendered could help international relations and reduce the risk of war.

If we all eat more plants and far less meat, we'd live longer healthier lives, make farming more sustainable, and help to mitigate climate change and resource scarcity leading to conflict.

If our cities become cooler and greener and better designed around coherent communities and energy-efficient public transport, then, again, that would reduce climate change impacts at the same time as allowing more physical activity and social interaction and support.

We need to tackle environmental design, making incidental physical activity easier, and rein in the food industry which is allowed to advertise and increase the consumption of cheap, unhealthy, calorie-dense, nutrition-poor foods. The battle over smoking is also not over as the tobacco industry has shifted its attention to low and middle income countries which should have the tobacco controls of rich nations. Remember that obesity and smoking swamp a lot else in terms of shortening lives and living longer sicker. For example, for every year you're obese you increase the risk of dying younger than you otherwise would by 1.5 per cent. For every year. Just add it up. Eliminating smoking would increase global life expectancy by more than two years in men and one year in women. That's the average diluted by the lower death rates of non-smokers. For individuals who smoke, the healthy life extension could be 20 years or more.

If new medical technologies were introduced more thoughtfully and their use controlled so we get the most value from them, then they'd be more affordable and less risky. The highest priority must be given to antibiotic misuse in human and animal health.

So you want to live younger longer? We know how. Just gotta do it.

And never forget, when prevention works, bad stuff doesn't happen.

Don't let the bastards get you down. I don't.

Acknowledgements

This book wouldn't have happened without the push from Gaby Naher, my utterly superb literary agent, ably supported by her team at Left Bank Literary. The person who thought this would be the right follow-on from my last book and was always there for support and guidance was Vanessa Radnidge, Head of Non-Fiction at Hachette. The editing process was made smooth by the efficient and highly skilled Karen Ward and Susin Chow, both of whom have judgement you can trust. The truly amazing Rosina Di Marzo is one of the best book publicists in the business. Eliza Harvey helped with research and, as always, added value, particularly with her critiques of ideas at the outset. My close colleagues at the ABC put up with a lot, especially my partners in *Coronacast*, Tegan Taylor and Will Ockenden. Tegan has also joined me on *The Health Report*, which is produced by the long-suffering Diane Dean. Joel Werner and Jonathan Webb in the ABC's Science Unit are unfailingly supportive as is the ABC's Managing Director, David Anderson. By the way, unfailingly supportive does not mean blind to my many flaws! I am grateful to Alan Lopez, Pat Jalland, Joy Damousi, Janet McCalman, David Bowtell, Penny Webb, Matthew Dunn, Jack Goldblatt, Ian Hickie, Liz Scott and Luigi Fontana for their advice, guidance and criticism. The responsibility for any errors in the interpretation of data is entirely mine. Hopefully there aren't too many. Finally, to

Katie and my children, Anna, Georgia and Jonathan, who keep me centred on what's important in life, you all know what you mean to me.

Notes

I was determined to make this book as strongly evidence based as possible while making the information as accessible as it can be to everyone. I didn't want to write an academic text with reference numbers. What follows are papers and sources which have informed the content of each section.

Introduction

Dunno about you but I intend to live forever

National Records of Scotland:
https://www.nrscotland.gov.uk/files//statistics/life-expectancy-in-
scotland/17-19/life-expectancy-17-19-report.pdf

Australian data:
https://www.abc.net.au/radionational/programs/healthreport/
median-age-of-death/13203336

PHIDU Torrens University: https://phidu.torrens.edu.au/pdf/2015-
onwards/factsheets/Summary%20of%20median%20age%20
at%20death-Australia.pdf

What is this staying young thing?

Jones OR, Vaupel JW. 'Senescence is not inevitable', *Biogerontology*. 2017 Dec; 18(6): 965–971. doi: 10.1007/s10522-017-9727-3. Epub 2017 Aug 28. PMID: 28849291; PMCID: PMC5743229

Malone JC, Liu SR, Vaillant GE, Rentz DM, Waldinger RJ. 'Midlife Eriksonian psychosocial development: Setting the stage for late-life cognitive and emotional health', *Dev Psychol*. 2016 Mar; 52(3): 496–508. doi: 10.1037/a0039875. Epub 2015 Nov 9. PMID: 26551530; PMCID: PMC5398200

Vaillant GE, Milofsky E. 'Natural history of male psychological health: IX. Empirical evidence for Erikson's model of the life cycle', *Am J Psychiatry.* 1980 Nov; 137(11): 1348–59

Blatný M, Millová K, Jelínek M, et al. 'Personality Predictors of Midlife Generativity: A Longitudinal Study', *J Adult Dev.* 2019; 26, 219–231. https://doi.org/10.1007/s10804-018-9323-z

Peterson BE, Klohnen EC. 'Realization of generativity in two samples of women at midlife', *Psychol Aging.* 1995 Mar; 10(1): 20–9. doi: 10.1037//0882-7974.10.1.20. PMID: 7779312

Bellingtier JA, Neupert SD. 'Feeling Young and in Control: Daily Control Beliefs Are Associated With Younger Subjective Ages', *J Gerontol B Psychol Sci Soc Sci.* 2020 Apr 16; 75(5): e13–e17. doi: 10.1093/geronb/gbz015. PMID: 30873557

Bellingtier JA, Rupprecht FS, Neupert SD, Lang FR. 'Daily experiences of subjective age discordance and well-being', *Psychol Aging.* 2021 Jul 22. doi: 10.1037/pag0000621. Epub ahead of print. PMID: 34291961

Kotter-Grühn D, Neupert SD, Stephan Y. 'Feeling old today? Daily health, stressors, and affect explain day-to-day variability in subjective age', *Psychol Health.* 2015; 30(12): 1470–85. doi: 10.1080/08870446.2015.1061130. Epub 2015 Jul 6. PMID: 26066614

The Book of Life

Herskind AM, McGue M, Holm NV, Sørensen TI, Harvald B, Vaupel JW. 'The heritability of human longevity: a population-based study of 2872 Danish twin pairs born 1870–1900', *Hum Genet.* 1996 Mar; 97(3): 319–23. doi: 10.1007/BF02185763. PMID: 8786073

Andersen SL, Sun JX, Sebastiani P, Huntly J, Gass JD, Feldman L, Bae H, Christiansen L, Perls TT. 'Personality factors in the Long Life Family Study', *J Gerontol B Psychol Sci Soc Sci.* 2013 Sep; 68(5): 739–49. doi: 10.1093/geronb/gbs117. Epub 2012 Dec 28. PMID: 23275497; PMCID: PMC3744045

https://www.abc.net.au/radionational/programs/healthreport/centenarian-study/3556620

Meredith HV. 'Finding from Asia, Australia, Europe, and North America on secular change in mean height of children, youths, and young adults', *Am J Phys Anthropol.* 1976 Mar; 44(2): 315–25. doi: 10.1002/ajpa.1330440214. PMID: 1258988

Petrova K, Nevarez MD, Rice J, et al. 'Coherence Between Feelings and Heart Rate: Links to Early Adversity and Responses to Stress', *Affec Sci.* 2021; 2: 1–13. https://doi.org/10.1007/s42761-020-00027-5

What really, really old people can teach us

https://www.pewresearch.org/fact-tank/2016/04/21/worlds-centenarian-population-projected-to-grow-eightfold-by-2050/

Wilson T, Terblanche W. 'New estimates of Australia's centenarian population', *Int J Popul Data Sci.* 2018 Jun 20; 3(1): 447. doi: 10.23889/ijpds.v3i1.447. PMID: 32935007; PMCID: PMC7299471

https://www.aihw.gov.au/reports/life-expectancy-death/deaths-in-australia/contents/life-expectancy

https://www.bumc.bu.edu/centenarian/

Sebastiani P, Solovieff N, Dewan AT, Walsh KM, Puca A, Hartley SW, Melista E, Andersen S, Dworkis DA, Wilk JB, Myers RH, Steinberg MH, Montano M, Baldwin CT, Hoh J, Perls TT. 'Genetic signatures of exceptional longevity in humans', *PLoS One.* 2012; 7(1): e29848. doi: 10.1371/journal.pone.0029848. Epub 2012 Jan 18. PMID: 22279548; PMCID: PMC3261167

Sebastiani P, Bae H, Sun FX, Andersen SL, Daw EW, Malovini A, Kojima T, Hirose N, Schupf N, Puca A, Perls TT. 'Meta-analysis of genetic variants associated with human exceptional longevity', *Aging* (Albany NY). 2013 Sep; 5(9): 653–61. doi: 10.18632/aging.100594. PMID: 24244950; PMCID: PMC3808698

Herskind AM, McGue M, Holm NV, Sørensen TI, Harvald B, Vaupel JW. 'The heritability of human longevity: a population-based study of 2872 Danish twin pairs born 1870–1900', *Hum Genet.* 1996 Mar; 97(3): 319–23. doi: 10.1007/BF02185763. PMID: 8786073

Shan Z, Rehm CD, Rogers G, et al. 'Trends in Dietary Carbohydrate, Protein, and Fat Intake and Diet Quality Among US Adults,

1999–2016', *JAMA*. 2019; 322(12): 1178–1187. doi:10.1001/
jama.2019.13771

Part 1 – Sweat the big stuff

Fontana L, Fasano A, Chong YS, Vineis P, Willett WC.
'Transdisciplinary research and clinical priorities for better
health', *PLoS Med*. 2021; 18(7): e1003699. https://doi.org/10.1371/
journal. pmed.1003699

https://www.worldometers.info/demographics/life-
expectancy/#countries-ranked-by-life-expectancy

https://www.statista.com/statistics/236541/per-capita-health-
expenditure-by-country/

https://www.worldometers.info/gdp/gdp-per-capita/

https://worldpopulationreview.com/country-rankings/income-
inequality-by-country

http://hdr.undp.org/en/content/human-development-index-hdi

Human Development Indices and Indicators 2018 Statistical Update.
United Nations Development Programme

http://hdr.undp.org/sites/default/files/2018_human_development_
statistical_update.pdf

García JL, Heckman JJ. 'Early childhood education and life-cycle
health', *Health Econ*. 2020 Sep 4; doi: 10.1002/hec.4148. Epub
ahead of print. PMID: 32885902; PMCID: PMC7930163

Lelieveld J, Pozzer A, Pöschl U, Fnais M, Haines A, Münzel T. 'Loss of
life expectancy from air pollution compared to other risk factors:
a worldwide perspective', *Cardiovascular Research*. 2020 Sep 1;
volume 116, issue 11, pp. 1910–1917. https://doi.org/10.1093/cvr/
cvaa025

Caldwell JC. 'Routes to Low Mortality in Poor Countries', *Population
and Development Review* (Population Council, Wiley). 1986;
volume 12, no. 2, pp. 171–220. https://doi.org/10.2307/1973108

GBD 2015 Mortality and Causes of Death Collaborators. 'Global,
regional, and national life expectancy, all-cause mortality, and
cause-specific mortality for 249 causes of death, 1980–2015: a
systematic analysis for the Global Burden of Disease Study 2015',

Lancet. 2016 Oct 8; 388(10053): 1459–1544. doi: 10.1016/S0140-6736(16)31012-1. Erratum in: *Lancet.* 2017 Jan 7; 389(10064): e1. PMID: 27733281; PMCID: PMC5388903

GBD 2013 DALYs and HALE Collaborators, Murray CJ, et al. 'Global, regional, and national disability-adjusted life years (DALYs) for 306 diseases and injuries and healthy life expectancy (HALE) for 188 countries, 1990–2013: quantifying the epidemiological transition', *Lancet.* 2015 Nov 28; 386(10009): 2145–91. doi: 10.1016/S0140-6736(15)61340-X. Epub 2015 Aug 28. PMID: 26321261; PMCID: PMC4673910

Granados JA. 'Health at advanced age: social inequality and other factors potentially impacting longevity in nine high-income countries', *Maturitas.* 2013 Feb; 74(2): 137–47. doi: 10.1016/j.maturitas.2012.11.013. Epub 2012 Dec 28. PMID: 23276601

The Glasgow Effect – young lives matter

Cowley J, Kiely J, Collins D. 'Unravelling the Glasgow effect: The relationship between accumulative bio-psychosocial stress, stress reactivity and Scotland's health problems', *Prev Med Rep.* 2016 Aug 3; 4: 370–5. doi: 10.1016/j.pmedr.2016.08.004. PMID: 27512652; PMCID: PMC4979043

With Sir Harry Burns: https://www.abc.net.au/radionational/programs/healthreport/unravelling-the-glasgow-effect/10392744

What the Taliban know

Caldwell JC. 'Routes to Low Mortality in Poor Countries', *Population and Development Review* (Population Council, Wiley). 1986; volume 12, no. 2, pp. 171–220. https://doi.org/10.2307/1973108

Lutz W, Kebede E. 'Education and Health: Redrawing the Preston Curve', *Popul Dev Rev.* 2018 Jun; 44(2): 343–361. doi: 10.1111/padr.12141. Epub 2018 Apr 14. PMID: 29937609; PMCID: PMC6001628

Lutz W, Samir KC. 'Global human capital: integrating education and population', *Science.* 2011 Jul 29; 333(6042): 587–92. doi: 10.1126/science.1206964. PMID: 21798940

Lutz W, Crespo Cuaresma J, Kebede E, Prskawetz A, Sanderson WC, Striessnig E. 'Education rather than age structure brings demographic dividend', *Proc Natl Acad Sci USA*. 2019 Jun 25; 116(26): 12798–12803. doi: 10.1073/pnas.1820362116. Epub 2019 Jun 10. PMID: 31182606; PMCID: PMC6600906

Preston SH. 'The changing relation between mortality and level of economic development. 1975', *Bull World Health Organ*. 2003; 81(11): 833–41. Epub 2004 Jan 20. PMID: 14758412; PMCID: PMC2572360

McKeown T, Record RG. 'Reasons for the decline of mortality in England and Wales during the nineteenth century', *Population Studies*. 1962; 16: 2, 94–122. doi: 10.1080/00324728.1962.10414870

Smith FB. *The retreat of tuberculosis 1850–1950*. 1988. Croom Helm: London

Fairchild AL, Oppenheimer GM. 'Program in the History of Public Health and Medicine', Columbia School of Public Health, New York City, NY 10032-2625, USA

Fairchild AL, Oppenheimer GM. 'Public health nihilism vs pragmatism: history, politics, and the control of tuberculosis', *American Journal of Public Health*. 1998 July 1; 88, no. 7, pp. 1105–1117. https://doi.org/10.2105/AJPH.88.7.1105 PMID: 9663166

Ramakrishnan T, Chandrasekhar P. 'The control of tuberculosis: a continuous game of snakes and ladders', *J Biosci*. 1991; 24: 143–152. https://doi.org/10.1007/BF02941194

Kustanto A. 'The Role of Socioeconomic and Environmental Factors on the Number of Tuberculosis Cases in Indonesia', *Jurnal Ekonomi Pembangunan*. 2020 Dec 5; volume 18 (2): 129–146. Available at SSRN: https://ssrn.com/abstract=3745292

Mind you

Wahlbeck K, Westman J, Nordentoft M, Gissler M, Laursen T. 'Outcomes of Nordic mental health systems: Life expectancy of patients with mental disorders', *British Journal of Psychiatry*. 2011; 199(6): 453–458. doi:10.1192/bjp.bp.110.085100

Harris C, Barraclough B. 'Excess mortality of mental disorder', *British Journal of Psychiatry*. 1998; 173(1): 11–53. doi:10.1192/bjp.173.1.11

Patton G. 'Mortality in eating disorders', *Psychological Medicine*. 1988; 18(4): 947–951. doi:10.1017/S0033291700009879

Doering LV, Moser DK, Riegel B, McKinley S, Davidson P, Baker H, Meischke H, Dracup K. 'Persistent comorbid symptoms of depression and anxiety predict mortality in heart disease', *Int J Cardiol*. 2010 Nov 19; 145(2): 188–192. doi: 10.1016/j.ijcard.2009.05.025. Epub 2009 Jun 2. PMID: 19493579; PMCID: PMC2998562

Plana-Ripoll O, Pedersen CB, Agerbo E, Holtz Y, Erlangsen A, Canudas-Romo V, Laursen TM. 'A comprehensive analysis of mortality-related health metrics associated with mental disorders: a nationwide, register-based cohort study', *Lancet*. 2019; doi:10.1016/S0140-6736(19)32316-5

Get out of those genes

https://lynchsyndrome.org.au/the-facts

Petrucelli N, Daly MB, Pal T. 'BRCA1- and BRCA2-Associated Hereditary Breast and Ovarian Cancer', 1998 Sep 4 [Updated 2016 Dec 15]. In: Adam MP, Ardinger HH, Pagon RA, et al (eds). GeneReviews® [Internet]. University of Washington: Seattle, WA. 1993–2021

https://www.canceraustralia.gov.au/sites/default/files/publications/nbocc-bog-2010-web-a4-printable_504af02a673fd.pdf

Anggraeni TD, Al Fattah AN, Surya R. 'Prophylactic salpingectomy and ovarian cancer: An evidence-based analysis', *South Asian J Cancer*. 2018 Jan–Mar; 7(1): 42–45. doi: 10.4103/sajc.sajc_187_17. PMID: 29600234; PMCID: PMC5865096

Kotsopoulos J, Narod SA. 'Prophylactic salpingectomy for the prevention of ovarian cancer: Who should we target?', *Int J Cancer*. 2020 Sep 1; 147(5): 1245–1251. doi: 10.1002/ijc.32916. Epub 2020 Feb 29. PMID: 32037528

Scheuner M, Setodji C, Pankow J, et al. 'Relation of familial patterns of coronary heart disease, stroke, and diabetes to subclinical atherosclerosis: the multi-ethnic study of atherosclerosis', *Genet Med*. 2008; 10: 879–887. https://doi.org/10.1097/GIM.0b013e31818e639b

https://www.victorchang.edu.au/congenital-heart-disease

https://thefhfoundation.org/familial-hypercholesterolemia/what-is-familial-hypercholesterolemia

Kirke A, Watts GF, Emery J. 'Detecting familial hypercholesterolaemia in general practice', *Aust Fam Physician.* 2012 Dec; 41(12): 965–8. PMID: 23210121

http://www.heartregistry.org.au/patients-families/genetic-heart-diseases/familial-dilated-cardiomyopathy/

Prostate cancer risk:

Li S, Silvestri V, et al. 'Cancer Risks Associated With BRCA1 and BRCA2 Pathogenic Variants', *J Clin Oncol.* 2022 Jan 25; JCO2102112. doi: 10.1200/JCO.21.02112. Epub ahead of print. PMID: 35077220

Cancer testing:

https://www.qimrberghofer.edu.au/pathwaysStudy/

Is what you see what you get and biological age

Christensen K, Thinggaard M. et al. 'Perceived age as clinically useful biomarker of ageing: cohort study', University of Southern Denmark. https://www.bmj.com/content/339/bmj.b5262

Low E, Alimohammadiha G, Smith LA, Costello LF, Przyborski SA, von Zglinicki T, Miwa S. 'How good is the evidence that cellular senescence causes skin ageing?', *Ageing Res Rev.* 2021 Nov; 71: 101456. doi: 10.1016/j.arr.2021.101456. Epub 2021 Sep 3. PMID: 34487917; PMCID: PMC8524668

Davies JMS, Cillard J, Friguet B, et al. 'The Oxygen Paradox, the French Paradox, and age-related diseases', *Geroscience.* 2017; 39(5–6): 499–550. doi:10.1007/s11357-017-0002-y

Rivas JM, Ullrich SE. 'Systemic suppression of delayed-type hypersensitivity by supernatants from UV-irradiated keratinocytes. An essential role for keratinocyte-derived IL-10', *J Immunol.* 1992 Dec 15; 149(12): 3865–71. PMID: 1460278

Skopelja-Gardner S, Tai J, Sun X, Tanaka L, Kuchenbecker JA, Snyder JM, Kubes P, Mustelin T, Elkon KB. 'Acute skin exposure to ultraviolet light triggers neutrophil-mediated kidney inflammation', *Proc Natl Acad Sci USA*. 2021 Jan 19; 118(3): e2019097118. doi: 10.1073/pnas.2019097118. PMID: 33397815; PMCID: PMC7826360

Moskalev A. 'The challenges of estimating biological age', *Elife*. 2020 Feb 11; 9: e54969. doi: 10.7554/eLife.54969. PMID: 32041685; PMCID: PMC7012619

Jylhävä J, Pedersen NL, Hägg S. 'Biological Age Predictors', *EBioMedicine*. 2017 Jul; 21: 29–36. doi: 10.1016/j.ebiom.2017.03.046. Epub 2017 Apr 1. PMID: 28396265; PMCID: PMC5514388

The balance thing

López-Otín C, Kroemer G. 'Hallmarks of Health', *Cell*. 2021 Jan 7; 184(1): 33–63. doi: 10.1016/j.cell.2020.11.034. Epub 2020 Dec 18. Erratum in: *Cell*. 2021 Apr 1; 184(7): 1929–1939. PMID: 33340459

Tower J. 'Programmed cell death in aging', *Ageing Res Rev*. 2015 Sep; 23(Pt A): 90–100. doi: 10.1016/j.arr.2015.04.002. Epub 2015 Apr 8. PMID: 25862945; PMCID: PMC4480161

Pomatto LCD, Davies KJA. 'The role of declining adaptive homeostasis in ageing', *J Physiol*. 2017 Dec 15; 595(24): 7275–7309. doi: 10.1113/JP275072. Epub 2017 Nov 21. PMID: 29028112; PMCID: PMC5730851

Pomatto LCD, Sun PY, Davies KJA. 'To adapt or not to adapt: Consequences of declining adaptive homeostasis and proteostasis with age', *Mech Ageing Dev*. 2019 Jan; 177: 80–87. doi: 10.1016/j.mad.2018.05.006. Epub 2018 May 17. PMID: 29778759; PMCID: PMC6240408

Where's reverse on the human gearshift?

Colchero F, Aburto JM, Archie EA, et al. 'The long lives of primates and the "invariant rate of ageing" hypothesis', *Nat Commun*. 2021; 12; 3666. https://doi.org/10.1038/s41467-021-23894-3

Lopez AD, Adair T. 'Is the long-term decline in cardiovascular-disease mortality in high-income countries over? Evidence from national vital statistics', *Int J Epidemiol*. 2019 Dec 1; 48(6): 1815–1823. doi: 10.1093/ije/dyz143. PMID: 31378814 van Raalte AA, Sasson I, Martikainen P. 'The case for monitoring life-span inequality', *Science*. 2018 Nov 30; 362(6418): 1002–1004. doi: 10.1126/science.aau5811. PMID: 30498117

Oeppen J, Vaupel JW. 'Demography. Broken limits to life expectancy', *Science*. 2002 May 10; 296(5570): 1029–31. doi: 10.1126/science.1069675. PMID: 12004104

Zuo W, Jiang S, Guo Z, Feldman MW, Tuljapurkar S. 'Advancing front of old-age human survival', *Proc Natl Acad Sci USA*. 2018 Oct 30; 115(44): 11209–11214. doi: 10.1073/pnas.1812337115. Epub 2018 Oct 16. PMID: 30327342; PMCID: PMC6217443

Aburto JM, Villavicencio F, Basellini U, Kjærgaard S, Vaupel JW. 'Dynamics of life expectancy and life span equality', *Proc Natl Acad Sci USA*. 2020 Mar 10; 117(10): 5250–5259. doi: 10.1073/pnas.1915884117. Epub 2020 Feb 24. PMID: 32094193; PMCID: PMC7071894

Vaupel JW, Villavicencio F, Bergeron-Boucher MP. 'Demographic perspectives on the rise of longevity', *Proc Natl Acad Sci USA*. 2021 Mar 2; 118(9): e2019536118. doi: 10.1073/pnas.2019536118. PMID: 33571137; PMCID: PMC7936303

https://www.soa.org/globalassets/assets/Files/Research/Projects/research-2016-06-ltc-morbidity-improvement.pdf

Rejuvenation is a thing

Conboy IM, Conboy MJ, Wagers AJ, Girma ER, Weissman IL, Rando TA. 'Rejuvenation of aged progenitor cells by exposure to a young systemic environment', *Nature*. 2005 Feb 17; 433(7027): 760–4. doi: 10.1038/nature03260. PMID: 15716955

Hofmann B. 'Young Blood Rejuvenates Old Bodies: A Call for Reflection when Moving from Mice to Men', *Transfus Med Hemother*. 2018 Jan; 45(1): 67–71. doi: 10.1159/000481828. Epub 2018 Jan 3. PMID: 29593463; PMCID: PMC5836258

Villeda S, Plambeck K, Middeldorp J, et al. 'Young blood reverses age-related impairments in cognitive function and synaptic plasticity in mice', *Nat Med*. 2014; 20: 659–66. https://doi.org/10.1038/nm.3569

Scudellari M. 'Ageing research: Blood to blood', *Nature*. 2015; 517: 426–429. https://doi.org/10.1038/517426a

Rebo J, Mehdipour M, Gathwala R, Causey K, Liu Y, Conboy MJ, Conboy IM. 'A single heterochronic blood exchange reveals rapid inhibition of multiple tissues by old blood', *Nat Commun*. 2016; 7: 13363. doi: 10.1038/ncomms13363

Mehdipour M, Skinner C, Wong N, Lieb M, Liu C, Etienne J, Kato C, Kiprov D, Conboy MJ, Conboy IM. 'Rejuvenation of three germ layers tissues by exchanging old blood plasma with saline-albumin', *Aging* (Albany NY). 2020; 12: 8790–819. doi: 10.18632/aging.103418

Pandika M. 'Looking to Young Blood to Treat the Diseases of Aging', *ACS Cent Sci*. 2019 Sep 25; 5(9): 1481–1484. doi: 10.1021/acscentsci.9b00902. Epub 2019 Sep 13. PMID: 31572771; PMCID: PMC6764071

Elabd C, Cousin W, Upadhyayula P, et al. 'Oxytocin is an age-specific circulating hormone that is necessary for muscle maintenance and regeneration', *Nat Commun*. 2014; 5: 4082. https://doi.org/10.1038/ncomms5082

Conboy IM, Rando TA. 'Heterochronic parabiosis for the study of the effects of aging on stem cells and their niches', *Cell Cycle*. 2012; 11: 12, 2260–2267. doi: 10.4161/cc.20437

Rebo J, Mehdipour M, Gathwala R, Causey K, Liu Y, Conboy MJ, Conboy IM. 'A single heterochronic blood exchange reveals rapid inhibition of multiple tissues by old blood', *Nat Commun*. 2016; 7: 13363. https://doi.org/10.1038/ncomms13363 [PubMed]

Mehdipour M, Etienne J, Chen CC, Gathwala R, Rehman M, Kato C, Liu C, Liu Y, Zuo Y, Conboy MJ, Conboy IM. 'Rejuvenation of brain, liver and muscle by simultaneous pharmacological modulation of two signaling determinants, that change in opposite directions with age', *Aging* (Albany NY). 2019 Aug 15; 11(15): 5628–5645. doi: 10.18632/aging.102148. Epub 2019 Aug 15. PMID: 31422380; PMCID: PMC6710051

Villeda SA, Luo J, Mosher KI, Zou B, Britschgi M, Bieri G, Stan TM, Fainberg N, Ding Z, Eggel A, Lucin KM, Czirr E, Park JS, et al.

'The ageing systemic milieu negatively regulates neurogenesis and cognitive function', *Nature*. 2011; 477: 90–94. https://doi.org/10.1038/nature10357 [PubMed]

https://newsnetwork.mayoclinic.org/discussion/mayo-clinic-discovers-high-intensity-aerobic-training-can-reverse-aging-processes-in-adults/

Robinson MM, Dasari S, Konopka AR, Johnson ML, Manjunatha S, Esponda RR, Carter RE, Lanza IR, Nair KS. 'Enhanced Protein Translation Underlies Improved Metabolic and Physical Adaptations to Different Exercise Training Modes in Young and Old Humans', *Cell Metab*. 2017 Mar 7; 25(3): 581–592. doi: 10.1016/j.cmet.2017.02.009. PMID: 28273480; PMCID: PMC5423095

Ruegsegger GN, Vanderboom PM, Dasari S, Klaus KA, Kabiraj P, McCarthy CB, Lucchinetti CF, Nair KS. 'Exercise and metformin counteract altered mitochondrial function in the insulin-resistant brain', *JCI Insight*. 2019 Sep 19; 4(18): e130681. doi: 10.1172/jci.insight.130681. PMID: 31534057; PMCID: PMC6795285

Nair KS. 'Aging muscle', *Am J Clin Nutr*. 2005 May; 81(5): 953–63. doi: 10.1093/ajcn/81.5.953. PMID: 15883415

Koh JH, Johnson ML, Dasari S, LeBrasseur NK, Vuckovic I, Henderson GC, Cooper SA, Manjunatha S, Ruegsegger GN, Shulman GI, Lanza IR, Nair KS. 'TFAM Enhances Fat Oxidation and Attenuates High-Fat Diet-Induced Insulin Resistance in Skeletal Muscle', *Diabetes*. 2019 Aug; 68(8): 1552–1564. doi: 10.2337/db19-0088. Epub 2019 May 14. Erratum in: *Diabetes*. 2020 Aug; 69(8): 1854. PMID: 31088855; PMCID: PMC6692815

Boada M, López OL, Olazarán J, Núñez L, Pfeffer M, Paricio M, Lorites J, Piñol-Ripoll G, Gámez JE, Anaya F, Kiprov D, Lima J, Grifols C, Torres M, Costa M, Bozzo J, Szczepiorkowski ZM, Hendrix S, Páez A. 'A randomized, controlled clinical trial of plasma exchange with albumin replacement for Alzheimer's disease: Primary results of the AMBAR Study', *Alzheimers*

Dement. 2020 Oct; 16(10): 1412–1425. doi: 10.1002/alz.12137. Epub 2020 Jul 27. PMID: 32715623; PMCID: PMC7984263

Mehdipour M, Skinner C, Wong N, Lieb M, Liu C, Etienne J, Kato C, Kiprov D, Conboy MJ, Conboy IM. 'Rejuvenation of three germ layers tissues by exchanging old blood plasma with saline-albumin', *Aging* (Albany NY). 2020 May 30; 12(10): 8790–8819. doi: 10.18632/aging.103418. Epub 2020 May 30. PMID: 32474458; PMCID: PMC7288913

Baker D, Childs B, Durik M, et al. 'Naturally occurring p16Ink4a-positive cells shorten healthy lifespan', *Nature.* 2016; 530: 184–189. https://doi.org/10.1038/nature16932

Jayarajan J, Milsom MD. 'The role of the stem cell epigenome in normal aging and rejuvenative therapy', *Human Molecular Genetics.* 2020 Oct 1; volume 29, issue R2, pp. R236–R247. https://doi.org/10.1093/hmg/ddaa167

Simpson DJ, Olova NN, Chandra T. 'Cellular reprogramming and epigenetic rejuvenation', *Clin Epigenet.* 2021; 13: 170. https://doi.org/10.1186/s13148-021-01158-7

Part 2 – Eating – not fasting – holds the secret

Green CL, Lamming DW, Fontana L. 'Molecular mechanisms of dietary restriction promoting health and longevity', *Nat Rev Mol Cell Biol.* 2022 Jan; 23(1): 56–73. doi: 10.1038/s41580-021-00411-4. Epub 2021 Sep 13. PMID: 34518687; PMCID: PMC8692439

Lowe DA, et al. 'Effects of time-restricted eating on weight loss and other metabolic parameters in women and men with overweight and obesity: the TREAT randomized clinical trial', *JAMA Intern Med.* 2020; 180: 1491–1499

Dhurandhar EJ, Dawson J, Alcorn A, et al. 'The effectiveness of breakfast recommendations on weight loss: a randomized controlled trial', *Am J Clin Nutr.* 2014; 100(2): 507–513. doi:10.3945/ajcn.114.089573

Farsijani S, Morais JA, Payette H, et al. 'Relation between mealtime distribution of protein intake and lean mass loss in free-living older adults of the NuAge study', *Am J Clin Nutr.* 2016; 104(3): 694–703. doi:10.3945/ajcn.116.130716

Mamerow MM, Mettler JA, English KL, et al. 'Dietary protein distribution positively influences 24-h muscle protein synthesis in healthy adults', *J Nutr.* 2014; 144(6): 876–880. doi:10.3945/jn.113.185280

Areta JL, Burke LM, Ross ML, et al. 'Timing and distribution of protein ingestion during prolonged recovery from resistance exercise alters myofibrillar protein synthesis', *J Physiol.* 2013; 591(9): 2319–2331. doi: 10.1113/jphysiol.2012.244897

Ryttig K, Flaten H, Rössner S. 'Long-term effects of a very low calorie diet (Nutrilett®) in obesity treatment. A prospective, randomized, comparison between VLCD and a hypocaloric diet+behavior modification and their combination', *Int J Obes.* 1997; 21: 574–579. https://doi.org/10.1038/sj.ijo.0800444

Moreno B, Crujeiras AB, Bellido D, et al. 'Obesity treatment by very low-calorie-ketogenic diet at two years: reduction in visceral fat and on the burden of disease', *Endocrine.* 2016; 54: 681–690. https://doi.org/10.1007/s12020-016-1050-2

Di Rosa C, Lattanzi G, Taylor SF, Manfrini S, Khazrai YM. 'Very low calorie ketogenic diets in overweight and obesity treatment: Effects on anthropometric parameters, body composition, satiety, lipid profile and microbiota', *Obes Res Clin Pract.* 2020 Nov–Dec; 14(6): 491–503. doi: 10.1016/j.orcp.2020.08.009. Epub 2020 Sep 9. PMID: 32919928

Castellana M, Conte E, Cignarelli A, et al. 'Efficacy and safety of very low calorie ketogenic diet (VLCKD) in patients with overweight and obesity: A systematic review and meta-analysis', *Rev Endocr Metab Disord.* 2020; 21: 5–16. https://doi.org/10.1007/s11154-019-09514-y

Muscogiuri G, El Ghoch M, Colao A, Hassapidou M, Yumuk V, Busetto L; Obesity Management Task Force (OMTF) of the European Association for the Study of Obesity (EASO). 'European Guidelines for Obesity Management in Adults with a Very Low-Calorie Ketogenic Diet: A Systematic Review and Meta-Analysis', *Obes Facts.* 2021; 14(2): 222–245. doi: 10.1159/000515381. Epub 2021 Apr 21. PMID: 33882506; PMCID: PMC8138199

Catterson JH, Khericha M, Dyson MC, Vincent AJ, Callard R, Haveron SM, Rajasingam A, Ahmad M, Partridge L. 'Short-Term, Intermittent Fasting Induces Long-Lasting Gut Health and TOR-Independent Lifespan Extension', *Curr Biol.* 2018 Jun 4; 28(11): 1714–1724. e4. doi: 10.1016/j.cub.2018.04.015. Epub 2018 May 17. PMID: 29779873; PMCID: PMC5988561

Wei M, Brandhorst S, Shelehchi M, Mirzaei H, Cheng CW, Budniak J, Groshen S, Mack WJ, Guen E, Di Biase S, Cohen P, Morgan TE, Dorff T, Hong K, Michalsen A, Laviano A, Longo VD. 'Fasting-mimicking diet and markers/risk factors for aging, diabetes, cancer, and cardiovascular disease', *Sci Transl Med.* 2017 Feb 15; 9(377): eaai8700. doi: 10.1126/scitranslmed.aai8700. PMID: 28202779; PMCID: PMC6816332

Brandhorst S, Choi IY, Wei M, Cheng CW, Sedrakyan S, Navarrete G, Dubeau L, Yap LP, Park R, Vinciguerra M, Di Biase S, Mirzaei H, Mirisola MG, Childress P, Ji L, Groshen S, Penna F, Odetti P, Perin L, Conti PS, Ikeno Y, Kennedy BK, Cohen P, Morgan TE, Dorff TB, Longo VD. 'A Periodic Diet that Mimics Fasting Promotes Multi-System Regeneration, Enhanced Cognitive Performance, and Healthspan', *Cell Metab.* 2015 Jul 7; 22(1): 86–99. doi: 10.1016/j.cmet.2015.05.012. Epub 2015 Jun 18. PMID: 26094889; PMCID: PMC4509734

Liao CY, Rikke BA, Johnson TE, Diaz V, Nelson JF. 'Genetic variation in the murine lifespan response to dietary restriction: from life extension to life shortening', *Aging Cell.* 2010 Feb; 9(1): 92–5. doi: 10.1111/j.1474-9726.2009.00533.x. Epub 2009 Oct 30. PMID: 19878144; PMCID: PMC3476836

Harper JM, Leathers CW, Austad SN. 'Does caloric restriction extend life in wild mice?' *Aging Cell.* 2006 Dec; 5(6): 441–9. doi: 10.1111/j.1474-9726.2006.00236.x. Epub 2006 Oct 27. PMID: 17054664; PMCID: PMC2923404

Colman RJ, Anderson RM, Johnson SC, Cruzen C, Simmons HA, Kemnitz JW, Weindruch R, Kastman EK, Kosmatka KJ, Beasley TM, Allison DB. 'Caloric Restriction Delays Disease Onset and Mortality in Rhesus Monkeys', *Science*. 2009 July 9; volume 324, issue 5937

Mattison JA, Roth GS, Beasley TM, Tilmont EM, Handy AM, Herbert RL, Longo DL, Allison DB, Young JE, Bryant M, Barnard D, Ward WF, Qi W, Ingram DK, de Cabo R. 'Impact of caloric restriction on health and survival in rhesus monkeys from the NIA study', *Nature*. 2012 Aug 30; volume 488, no. 7413

Austad S. 'Mixed results for dieting monkeys', *Nature*. 2012 Aug 30; volume 488, no. 7413

Mattison J, Colman R, Beasley T, et al. 'Caloric restriction improves health and survival of rhesus monkeys', *Nat Commun*. 2017; 8: 14063. https://doi.org/10.1038/ncomms14063

Kraus WE, Bhapkar M, Huffman KM, Pieper CF, Krupa Das S, Redman LM, Villareal DT, Rochon J, Roberts SB, Ravussin E, Holloszy JO, Fontana L; CALERIE Investigators. '2 years of calorie restriction and cardiometabolic risk (CALERIE): exploratory outcomes of a multicentre, phase 2, randomised controlled trial', *Lancet Diabetes Endocrinol*. 2019 Sep; 7(9): 673–683. doi: 10.1016/S2213-8587(19)30151-2. Epub 2019 Jul 11. PMID: 31303390; PMCID: PMC6707879

Thodis, Antonia. 'MEDiterranean ISlands-Australia Study: Greek Mediterranean Diet Pattern Adherence, Successful Aging and Associations in Greek Australian Island-Born Long-Term Migrants.' 2019. La Trobe University (PhD Thesis)

Goji berries, cider vinegar and magical thinking

Hempel J, Schädle CN, Sprenger J, Heller A, Carle R, Schweiggert RM. 'Ultrastructural deposition forms and bioaccessibility of carotenoids and carotenoid esters from goji berries (*Lycium barbarum L.*)', *Food Chem*. 2017 Mar 1; 218: 525–533. doi: 10.1016/j.foodchem.2016.09.065. Epub 2016 Sep 10. PMID: 27719945

Luo Y, Liu Y, Guo H, Fu H. 'Evaluation of the bioaccessibility of carotenoid esters from *Lycium barbarum L.* in nano-emulsions:

A kinetic approach', *Food Res Int.* 2020 Oct; 136: 109611. doi: 10.1016/j.foodres.2020.109611. Epub 2020 Aug 1. PMID: 32846631

Song MK, Roufogalis BD, Huang THW. 'Modulation of RAGE and the Downstream Targets of RAGE Signaling Cascades by Taurine in *Lycium Barbarum* (Goji Berry): Protection of Human Retinal Pigment Epithelial Barrier Function and its Potential Benefit in Diabetic Retinopathy', *J Diabetes Metab.* 2011; 2: 162. doi:10.4172/2155-6156.1000162

Launholt TL, Kristiansen CB, Hjorth P. 'Safety and side effects of apple vinegar intake and its effect on metabolic parameters and body weight: a systematic review', *Eur J Nutr.* 2020; 59: 2273–2289. https://doi.org/10.1007/s00394-020-02214-3

https://www.mordorintelligence.com/industry-reports/apple-cider-vinegar-market

Goyal A, Sharma V, Upadhyay N, Gill S, Sihag M. 'Flax and flaxseed oil: an ancient medicine & modern functional food', *J Food Sci Technol.* 2014 Sep; 51(9): 1633–53. doi: 10.1007/s13197-013-1247-9. Epub 2014 Jan 10. PMID: 25190822; PMCID: PMC4152533

Cheng C, Yu X, Huang F, Peng D, Chen H, Chen Y, Huang Q, Deng Q. 'Effect of different structural flaxseed lignans on the stability of flaxseed oil-in-water emulsion: An interfacial perspective', *Food Chem.* 2021 Apr 8; 357: 129522. doi: 10.1016/j.foodchem.2021.129522. Epub ahead of print. PMID: 33872871

Part 3 – Which pill and why?

Tome-Carneiro J, et al. 'Resveratrol and clinical trials: the crossroad from in vitro studies to human evidence', *Curr Pharm Des.* 2013; 19: 6064–6093

Berman AY, Motechin RA, Wiesenfeld MY, et al. 'The therapeutic potential of resveratrol: a review of clinical trials', *npj Precision Onc 1.* 2017; 35. https://doi.org/10.1038/s41698-017-0038-6

Khorshidi F, Poljak A, Liu Y, Lo JW, Crawford JD, Sachdev PS. 'Resveratrol: A "miracle" drug in neuropsychiatry or a cognitive enhancer for mice only? A systematic review and meta-analysis', *Ageing Res Rev.* 2021 Jan; 65: 101199. doi: 10.1016/j.arr.2020.101199. Epub 2020 Oct 22. PMID: 33303422 de Ligt M, Bergman M, Fuentes RM, Essers H, Moonen-Kornips E, Havekes B, Schrauwen-Hinderling VB, Schrauwen P. 'No effect of resveratrol supplementation after 6 months on insulin sensitivity in overweight adults: a randomized trial', *The American Journal of Clinical Nutrition*. 2020 Oct; volume 112, issue 4, pp. 1029–1038. https://doi.org/10.1093/ajcn/nqaa125

Chudzińska M, Rogowicz D, Wołowiec Ł, et al. 'Resveratrol and cardiovascular system—the unfulfilled hopes', *Ir J Med Sci*. 2021; 190: 981–986. https://doi.org/10.1007/s11845-020-02441-x

Huang CC, Liu CC, Tsao JP, Hsu CL, Cheng IS. 'Effects of Oral Resveratrol Supplementation on Glycogen Replenishment and Mitochondria Biogenesis in Exercised Human Skeletal Muscle', *Nutrients*. 2020 Dec 2; 12(12): 3721. doi: 10.3390/nu12123721. PMID: 33276518; PMCID: PMC7760965

Campbell JM, Bellman SM, Stephenson MD, Lisy K. 'Metformin reduces all-cause mortality and diseases of ageing independent of its effect on diabetes control: A systematic review and meta-analysis', *Ageing Res Rev*. 2017 Nov; 40: 31–44. doi: 10.1016/j. arr.2017.08.003. Epub 2017 Aug 10. PMID: 28802803

Samaras K, Makkar S, Crawford JD, Kochan NA, Wen W, Draper B, Trollor JN, Brodaty H, Sachdev PS. 'Metformin Use Is Associated With Slowed Cognitive Decline and Reduced Incident Dementia in Older Adults With Type 2 Diabetes: The Sydney Memory and Ageing Study', *Diabetes Care*. 2020 Nov; 43(11): 2691–2701. doi: 10.2337/dc20-0892. Epub 2020 Sep 23. PMID: 32967921

Imfeld P, Bodmer M, Jick SS, Meier CR. 'Metformin, other antidiabetic drugs, and risk of Alzheimer's disease: a population-based case-control study', *J Am Geriatr Soc*. 2012 May; 60(5): 916–21. doi: 10.1111/j.1532-5415.2012.03916.x. Epub 2012 Mar 28. PMID: 22458300

Martin-Montalvo A, Mercken EM, Mitchell SJ, Palacios HH, Mote PL, Scheibye-Knudsen M, Gomes AP, Ward TM, Minor RK, Blouin MJ, Schwab M, Pollak M, Zhang Y, Yu Y, Becker KG, Bohr VA, Ingram DK, Sinclair DA, Wolf NS, Spindler SR, Bernier M, de Cabo R. 'Metformin improves healthspan and lifespan in mice', *Nat Commun.* 2013; 4: 2192. doi: 10.1038/ncomms3192. PMID: 23900241; PMCID: PMC3736576

Glossmann HH, Lutz OMD. 'Metformin and Aging: A Review', *Gerontology.* 2019; 65(6): 581–590. doi: 10.1159/000502257. Epub 2019 Sep 13. PMID: 31522175

Braun B, Eze P, Stephens BR, Hagobian TA, Sharoff CG, Chipkin SR, Goldstein B. 'Impact of metformin on peak aerobic capacity', *Appl Physiol Nutr Metab.* 2008 Feb; 33(1): 61–7. doi: 10.1139/H07-144. PMID: 18347654

Long DE, Peck BD, Martz JL, Tuggle SC, Bush HM, McGwin G, Kern PA, Bamman MM, Peterson CA. 'Metformin to Augment Strength Training Effective Response in Seniors (MASTERS): study protocol for a randomized controlled trial', *Trials.* 2017 Apr 26; 18(1): 192. doi: 10.1186/s13063-017-1932-5. PMID: 28441958; PMCID: PMC5405504

Walton RG, Dungan CM, Long DE, Tuggle SC, Kosmac K, Peck BD, Bush HM, Villasante Tezanos AG, McGwin G, Windham ST, Ovalle F, Bamman MM, Kern PA, Peterson CA. 'Metformin blunts muscle hypertrophy in response to progressive resistance exercise training in older adults: A randomized, double-blind, placebo-controlled, multicenter trial: The MASTERS trial', *Aging Cell.* 2019 Dec; 18(6): e13039. doi: 10.1111/acel.13039. Epub 2019 Sep 26. Erratum in: *Aging Cell.* 2020 Mar; 19(3): e13098. PMID: 31557380; PMCID: PMC6826125

Tang GH, Satkunam M, Pond GR, Steinberg GR, Blandino G, Schünemann HJ, Muti P. 'Association of Metformin with Breast Cancer Incidence and Mortality in Patients with Type II Diabetes: A GRADE-Assessed Systematic Review and Meta-analysis', *Cancer Epidemiol Biomarkers Prev.* 2018 Jun; 27(6): 627–635. doi: 10.1158/1055-9965.EPI-17-0936. Epub 2018 Apr 4. PMID: 29618465

Farmer RE, Ford D, Forbes HJ, Chaturvedi N, Kaplan R, Smeeth L, Bhaskaran K. 'Metformin and cancer in type 2 diabetes: a systematic review and comprehensive bias evaluation',

International Journal of Epidemiology. 2017 Apr; volume 46, issue 2, pp. 728–744. https://doi.org/10.1093/ije/dyw275

Blagosklonny MV. 'Fasting and rapamycin: diabetes versus benevolent glucose intolerance', *Cell Death Dis*. 2019; 10: 607. https://doi.org/10.1038/s41419-019-1822-8

Bjedov I, Rallis C. 'The Target of Rapamycin Signalling Pathway in Ageing and Lifespan Regulation', *Genes*. 2020; 11(9): 1043. https://doi.org/10.3390/genes11091043

Sehgal SN, Baker H, Vézina C. 'Rapamycin (AY-22,989), a new antifungal antibiotic. II. Fermentation, isolation and characterization', *J Antibiot*. 1975; 28: 727–732

Sehgal SN. 'Sirolimus: Its discovery, biological properties, and mechanism of action', *Transplant Proc*. 2003; 35: S7–S14

Liu GY, Sabatini DM. 'mTOR at the nexus of nutrition, growth, ageing and disease', *Nat Rev Mol Cell Biol*. 2020; 21: 183–203

Fu J, Shao CJ, Chen FR, Ng HK, Chen ZP. 'Autophagy induced by valproic acid is associated with oxidative stress in glioma cell lines', *Neuro Oncol*. 2010 Apr; 12(4): 328–40. doi: 10.1093/neuonc/nop005. Epub 2009 Oct 15. PMID: 20308311; PMCID: PMC2940599

Motoi Y, Shimada K, Ishiguro K, Hattori N. 'Lithium and autophagy', *ACS Chem Neurosci*. 2014 Jun 18; 5(6): 434–42. doi: 10.1021/cn500056q. Epub 2014 Apr 30. PMID: 24738557; PMCID: PMC4063500

Mannick JB, Morris M, Hockey H-UP, Roma G, Beibel M, Kulmatycki K, Watkins M, Shavlakadze T, Zhou W, Quinn D, et al. 'TORC1 inhibition enhances immune function and reduces infections in the elderly', *Sci Transl Med*. 2018; 10: eaaq1564

Madeo F, Bauer MA, Carmona-Gutierrez D, Kroemer G. 'Spermidine: a physiological autophagy inducer acting as an anti-aging vitamin in humans?', *Autophagy*. 2019 Jan; 15(1): 165–168. doi: 10.1080/15548627.2018.1530929. Epub 2018 Oct 11. PMID: 30306826; PMCID: PMC6287690

Singh A, D'Amico D, Andreux PA, et al. 'Direct supplementation with Urolithin A overcomes limitations of dietary exposure and gut microbiome variability in healthy adults to achieve consistent levels across the population', *Eur J Clin Nutr.* 2021. https://doi.org/10.1038/s41430-021-00950-1

Admasu TD, Chaithanya Batchu K, Barardo D, Ng LF, Lam VYM, Xiao L, Cazenave-Gassiot A, Wenk MR, Tolwinski NS, Gruber J. 'Drug Synergy Slows Aging and Improves Healthspan through IGF and SREBP Lipid Signaling', *Dev Cell.* 2018 Oct 8; 47(1): 67–79, e5. doi: 10.1016/j.devcel.2018.09.001. Epub 2018 Sep 27. PMID: 30269951

More pills to sell you – NAD+ precursors

Connell NJ, Grevendonk L, Fealy CE, Moonen-Kornips E, Bruls YMH, Schrauwen-Hinderling VB, de Vogel J, Hageman R, Geurts J, Zapata-Perez R, Houtkooper RH, Havekes B, Hoeks J, Schrauwen P. 'NAD+ Precursor Supplementation With L-Tryptophan, Nicotinic Acid, and Nicotinamide Does Not Affect Mitochondrial Function or Skeletal Muscle Function in Physically Compromised Older Adults', *The Journal of Nutrition.* 2021 Oct; volume 151, issue 10, pp. 2917–2931. https://doi.org/10.1093/jn/nxab193

Martens CR, Denman BA, Mazzo MR, Armstrong ML, Reisdorph N, McQueen MB, Chonchol M, Seals DR. 'Chronic nicotinamide riboside supplementation is well-tolerated and elevates NAD+ in healthy middle-aged and older adults', *Nat Commun.* 2018 Mar 29; 9(1): 1286. doi: 10.1038/s41467-018-03421-7. PMID: 29599478; PMCID: PMC5876407

Remie CME, Roumans KHM, Moonen MPB, Connell NJ, Havekes B, Mevenkamp J, Lindeboom L, de Wit VHW, van de Weijer T, Aarts SABM, Lutgens E, Schomakers BV, Elfrink HL, Zapata-Pérez R, Houtkooper RH, Auwerx J, Hoeks J, Schrauwen-Hinderling VB, Phielix E, Schrauwen P. 'Nicotinamide riboside supplementation alters body composition and skeletal muscle acetylcarnitine concentrations in healthy obese humans', *Am J Clin Nutr.* 2020 Aug 1; 112(2): 413–426. doi: 10.1093/ajcn/nqaa072. PMID: 32320006; PMCID: PMC7398770

Dollerup OL, Christensen B, Svart M, Schmidt MS, Sulek K, Ringgaard S, Stodkilde-Jorgensen H, Moller N, Brenner C, Treebak JT, et al. 'A randomized placebo-controlled clinical trial of nicotinamide riboside in obese men: Safety, insulin-sensitivity, and lipid-mobilizing effects', *Am J Clin Nutr.* 2018; 108(2): 343–53

Hershberger K, Martin A, Hirschey M. 'Role of NAD+ and mitochondrial sirtuins in cardiac and renal diseases', *Nat Rev Nephrol.* 2017; 13: 213–225. https://doi.org/10.1038/nrneph.2017.5

Elhassan YS, Kluckova K, Fletcher RS, Schmidt MS, Garten A, Doig CL, Cartwright DM, Oakey L, Burley CV, Jenkinson N, et al. 'Nicotinamide riboside augments the aged human skeletal muscle NAD(+) metabolome and induces transcriptomic and antiinflammatory signatures', *Cell Rep.* 2019; 28(7): 1717–1728, e6

Cocktails, the Mediterranean diet and frugality may go together

Jennings A, Koch M, Bang C, Franke A, Lieb W, Cassidy A. 'Microbial Diversity and Abundance of Parabacteroides Mediate the Associations Between Higher Intake of Flavonoid-Rich Foods and Lower Blood Pressure', *Hypertension.* 2021 Sep; 78(4): 1016–1026. doi: 10.1161

Jennings A, et al. 'Mediterranean-Style Diet Improves Systolic Blood Pressure and Arterial Stiffness in Older Adults', *Hypertension.* 2019 Mar; 73(3): 578–586. doi: 10.1161

Substances that may save you from eating your veggies (not)

Yousefzadeh MJ, Zhu Y, McGowan SJ, Angelini L, Fuhrmann-Stroissnigg H, Xu M, Ling YY, Melos KI, Pirtskhalava T, Inman CL, McGuckian C, Wade EA, Kato JI, Grassi D, Wentworth M, Burd CE, Arriaga EA, Ladiges WL, Tchkonia T, Kirkland JL, Robbins PD, Niedernhofer LJ. 'Fisetin is a senotherapeutic that extends health and lifespan', *EBioMedicine.* 2018 Oct; 36: 18–28. doi: 10.1016/j.ebiom.2018.09.015. Epub 2018 Sep 29. PMID: 30279143; PMCID: PMC6197652

Ravula AR, Teegala SB, Kalakotla S, Pasangulapati JP, Perumal V, Boyina HK. 'Fisetin, potential flavonoid with multifarious targets for treating neurological disorders: An updated review',

Eur J Pharmacol. 2021 Nov 5; 910: 174492. doi: 10.1016/j. ejphar.2021.174492. Epub 2021 Sep 10. PMID: 34516952

Maher P. 'Preventing and Treating Neurological Disorders with the Flavonol Fisetin', *Brain Plast.* 2021 Feb 9; 6(2): 155–166. doi: 10.3233/BPL-200104. PMID: 33782648; PMCID: PMC7990461

Beking K, Vieira A. 'Flavonoid intake and disability-adjusted life years due to Alzheimer's and related dementias: a population-based study involving twenty-three developed countries', *Public Health Nutr.* 2010 Sep; 13(9): 1403–9. doi: 10.1017/S1368980009992990. Epub 2010 Jan 11. PMID: 20059796

Commenges D, Scotet V, Renaud S, Jacqmin-Gadda H, Barberger-Gateau P, Dartigues JF. 'Intake of flavonoids and risk of dementia', *Eur J Epidemiol.* 2000 Apr; 16(4): 357–63. doi: 10.1023/a:1007614613771. PMID: 10959944

Colman R, Tchkonia T, Pirtskhalava T, Giorgadze N, Prata L, Schaefer K, Kirkland J. 'Effect of Combined Dasatinib and Fisetin Treatment on Senescent Cell Clearance in Monkeys', *Innov Aging.* 2020 Dec 16; 4(Suppl 1): 131–2. doi: 10.1093/geroni/igaa057.432. PMCID: PMC7740648

Huang H, Liao D, Dong Y, Pu R. 'Effect of quercetin supplementation on plasma lipid profiles, blood pressure, and glucose levels: a systematic review and meta-analysis', *Nutr Rev.* 2020 Aug 1; 78(8): 615–626. doi: 10.1093/nutrit/nuz071. PMID: 31940027

Ren F, Reilly K, Kerry JP, Gaffney M, Hossain M, Rai DK. 'Higher Antioxidant Activity, Total Flavonols, and Specific Quercetin Glucosides in Two Different Onion (*Allium cepa L.*) Varieties Grown under Organic Production: Results from a 6-Year Field Study', *J Agric Food Chem.* 2017 Jun 28; 65(25): 5122–5132. doi: 10.1021/acs.jafc.7b01352. Epub 2017 Jun 14. Erratum in: *J Agric Food Chem.* 2019 Mar 13; 67(10): 3068. PMID: 28612608

Li N, Sun C, Zhou B, Xing H, Ma D, Chen G, Weng D. 'Low concentration of quercetin antagonizes the cytotoxic effects of anti-neoplastic drugs in ovarian cancer', *PLoS One.* 2014 Jul 7; 9(7): e100314. doi: 10.1371/journal.pone.0100314. PMID: 24999622; PMCID: PMC4085066

Kleemann R, Verschuren L, Morrison M, Zadelaar S, van Erk MJ, Wielinga PY, Kooistra T. 'Anti-inflammatory, anti-proliferative and anti-atherosclerotic effects of quercetin in human in vitro and in vivo models', *Atherosclerosis*. 2011 Sep; 218(1): 44–52. doi: 10.1016/j.atherosclerosis.2011.04.023. Epub 2011 May 5. PMID: 21601209

You don't want bad neighbours

van Deursen JM. 'The role of senescent cells in ageing', *Nature*. 2014 May 22; 509(7501): 439–46. doi: 10.1038/nature13193. PMID: 24848057; PMCID: PMC4214092

Gasek NS, Kuchel GA, Kirkland JL, et al. 'Strategies for targeting senescent cells in human disease', *Nat Aging*. 2021; 1: 870–879. https://doi.org/10.1038/s43587-021-00121-8

Part 4 – Outrunning the clock – staying young with exercise

Chakravarty EF, Hubert HB, Lingala VB, Fries JF. 'Reduced disability and mortality among aging runners: a 21-year longitudinal study', *Arch Intern Med*. 2008 Aug 11; 168(15): 1638–46

Lee DC, Brellenthin AG, Thompson PD, Sui X, Lee IM, Lavie CJ. 'Running as a Key Lifestyle Medicine for Longevity', *Prog Cardiovasc Dis*. 2017 June–July; 60(1): 45–55. doi: 10.1016/j. pcad.2017.03.005. Epub 2017 Mar 30. PMID: 28365296

Chen XK, Yi ZN, Wong GT, Hasan KMM, Kwan JS, Ma AC, Chang RC. 'Is exercise a senolytic medicine? A systematic review', *Aging Cell*. 2021 Jan; 20(1): e13294. doi: 10.1111/acel.13294. Epub 2020 Dec 30. PMID: 33378138; PMCID: PMC7811843

Englund DA, Sakamoto AE, Fritsche CM, Heeren AA, Zhang X, Kotajarvi BR, Lecy DR, Yousefzadeh MJ, Schafer MJ, White TA, Atkinson EJ, LeBrasseur NK. 'Exercise reduces circulating biomarkers of cellular senescence in humans', *Aging Cell*. 2021 Jul; 20(7): e13415. doi: 10.1111/acel.13415. Epub 2021 Jun 8. PMID: 34101960; PMCID: PMC8282238

López-Otín C, Blasco MA, Partridge L, Serrano M, Kroemer G. 'The hallmarks of aging', *Cell*. 2013 Jun 6; 153(6): 1194–217. doi: 10.1016/j.cell.2013.05.039. PMID: 23746838; PMCID: PMC3836174

Carapeto PV, Aguayo-Mazzucato C. 'Effects of exercise on cellular and tissue aging', *Aging* (Albany NY). 2021 May 13; 13(10): 14522–14543. doi: 10.18632/aging.203051. Epub 2021 May 13. PMID: 34001677; PMCID: PMC8202894

World Health Organization. 'Global health risks: mortality and burden of disease attributable to selected major risks'. 2009

Erickson KI, Leckie RL, Weinstein AM. 'Physical activity, fitness, and gray matter volume', *Neurobiol Aging.* 2014 Sep; 35 Suppl 2: S20–8. doi: 10.1016/j.neurobiolaging.2014.03.034. Epub 2014 May 14. PMID: 24952993; PMCID: PMC4094356

Fisher G, Brown AW, Bohan Brown MM, Alcorn A, Noles C, Winwood L, et al. 'High Intensity Interval- vs Moderate Intensity- Training for Improving Cardiometabolic Health in Overweight or Obese Males: A Randomized Controlled Trial', *PLoS ONE.* 2015; 10(10): e0138853. https://doi.org/10.1371/journal.pone.0138853

Wen CP, Wai JP, Tsai MK, Chen CH. 'Minimal amount of exercise to prolong life: to walk, to run, or just mix it up?', *J Am Coll Cardiol.* 2014 Aug 5; 64(5): 482–4. doi: 10.1016/j.jacc.2014.05.026. PMID: 25082582

Lee D, Pate RR, Lavie CJ, Sui X, Church TS, Blair SN. 'Leisure-time running reduces all-cause and cardiovascular mortality risk', *J Am Coll Cardiol.* 2014; 64: 472–481

Wen CP, Wai JP, Tsai MK, Yang YC, Cheng TY, Lee MC, Chan HT, Tsao CK, Tsai SP, Wu X. 'Minimum amount of physical activity for reduced mortality and extended life expectancy: a prospective cohort study', *Lancet.* 2011 Oct 1; 378(9798): 1244–53. doi: 10.1016/S0140-6736(11)60749-6. Epub 2011 Aug 16. PMID: 21846575

Paluch AE, Gabriel KP, Fulton JE, et al. 'Steps per Day and All-Cause Mortality in Middle-aged Adults in the Coronary Artery Risk Development in Young Adults Study', *JAMA Netw Open.* 2021; 4(9): e2124516. doi:10.1001/jamanetworkopen.2021.24516

Werner CM, Hecksteden A, Morsch A, Zundler J, Wegmann M, Kratzsch J, Thiery J, Hohl M, Bittenbring JT, Neumann F, Böhm M, Meyer T, Laufs U. 'Differential effects of endurance, interval, and resistance training on telomerase activity and telomere length in a randomized, controlled study', *Eur Heart J.* 2019 Jan 1; 40(1): 34–46. doi: 10.1093/eurheartj/ehy585. PMID: 30496493; PMCID: PMC6312574

Schnohr P, O'Keefe JH, Lavie CJ, Holtermann A, Lange P, Jensen GB, Marott JL. 'U-Shaped Association Between Duration of Sports Activities and Mortality: Copenhagen City Heart Study', *Mayo Clin Proc.* 2021 Dec; 96(12): 3012–3020. doi: 10.1016/j.mayocp.2021.05.028. Epub 2021 Aug 17. PMID: 34412854

Get a grip

Chan J, Lu YC, Yao MMS, et al. 'Correlation between hand grip strength and regional muscle mass in older Asian adults: an observational study', *BMC Geriatr.* 2022; 22: 206. https://doi.org/10.1186/s12877-022-02898-8

Parra-Soto S, Tumblety C, Ho FK, Pell JP, Celis-Morales C. 'Associations Between Relative Grip Strength and the Risk of 15 Cancer Sites', *Am J Prev Med.* 2022 Feb; 62(2): e87–e95. doi: 10.1016/j.amepre.2021.07.015. Epub 2021 Oct 20. PMID: 34686389

Part 5 – Bugs, bowels and hormones

Bian G, Gloor GB, Gong A, Jia C, Zhang W, Hu J, Zhang H, Zhang Y, Zhou Z, Zhang J, et al. 'The gut microbiota of healthy aged Chinese is similar to that of the healthy young', *mSphere.* 2017 Sep 27; 2(5): e00327–17. doi: 10.1128/mSphere.00327-17

Galkin F, et al. 'Human Gut Microbiome Aging Clock Based on Taxonomic Profiling and Deep Learning', *iScience.* 2020. doi.org/10.1016/j.isci.2020.101199

Nagpal R, Mainali R, Ahmadi S, Wang S, Singh R, Kavanagh K, Kitzman DW, Kushugulova A, Marotta F, Yadav H. 'Gut microbiome and aging: Physiological and mechanistic insights', *Nutr Healthy Aging.* 2018 June 15; 4(4): 267–285. doi: 10.3233/NHA-170030. PMID: 29951588; PMCID: PMC6004897

Biagi E, Candela M, Fairweather-Tait S, Franceschi C, Brigidi P. 'Aging of the human metaorganism: The microbial counterpart', *Age* (Dordr). 2012; 34(1): 247–67. [5]

Keller JM, Surawicz CM. 'Clostridium difficile infection in the elderly', *Clin Geriatr Med.* 2014; 30(1): 79–93

Zapata HJ, Quagliarello VJ. 'The microbiota and microbiome in aging: Potential implications in health and age-related diseases', *J Am Geriatr Soc.* 2015; 63(4): 776–81

Buford TW. '(Dis) Trust your gut: The gut microbiome in age-related inflammation, health, and disease', *Microbiome.* 2017; 5(80): 1–11

Ghosh TS, Rampelli S, Jeffery IB, et al. 'Mediterranean diet intervention alters the gut microbiome in older people reducing frailty and improving health status: the NU-AGE 1-year dietary intervention across five European countries', *Gut.* 2020; 69: 1218–1228

Berendsen AAM, van de Rest O, Feskens EJM, Santoro A, Ostan R, Pietruszka B, Brzozowska A, Stelmaszczyk-Kusz A, Jennings A, Gillings R, Cassidy A, Caille A, Caumon E, Malpuech-Brugere C, Franceschi C, de Groot LCPGM. 'Changes in Dietary Intake and Adherence to the NU-AGE Diet Following a One-Year Dietary Intervention among European Older Adults – Results of the NU-AGE Randomized Trial', *Nutrients.* 2018 Dec 4; 10(12): 1905. doi: 10.3390/nu10121905. PMID: 30518044; PMCID: PMC6315357

Tran TTT, Cousin FJ, Lynch DB, et al. 'Prebiotic supplementation in frail older people affects specific gut microbiota taxa but not global diversity', *Microbiome.* 2019; 7: 39

Meslier V, Laiola M, Roager HM, De Filippis F, Roume H, Quinquis B, Giacco R, Mennella I, Ferracane R, Pons N, Pasolli E, Rivellese A, Dragsted LO, Vitaglione P, Ehrlich SD, Ercolini D. 'Mediterranean diet intervention in overweight and obese subjects lowers plasma cholesterol and causes changes in the gut microbiome and metabolome independently of energy intake', *Gut.* 2020 July; 69(7): 1258–1268. doi: 10.1136/gutjnl-2019-320438. Epub 2020 Feb 19. PMID: 32075887; PMCID: PMC7306983

Zaneveld JR, McMinds R, Vega Thurber R. 'Stress and stability: applying the Anna Karenina principle to animal microbiomes', *Nat Microbiol.* 2017; 2: 17121

Ghosh TS, Das M, Jeffery IB, O'Toole PW. 'Adjusting for age improves identification of gut microbiome alterations in multiple diseases', *Elife*. 2020 Mar 11; 9: e50240. doi: 10.7554/eLife.50240. PMID: 32159510; PMCID: PMC7065848

Maslowski KM, Vieira AT, Ng A, Kranich J, Sierro F, Yu D, Schilter HC, Rolph MS, Mackay F, Artis D, Xavier RJ, Teixeira MM, Mackay CR. 'Regulation of inflammatory responses by gut microbiota and chemoattractant receptor GPR43', *Nature*. 2009; 461(7268): 1282–6

De Smet R, Van Kaer J, Van Vlem B, De Cubber A, Brunet P, Lameire N, Vanholder R. 'Toxicity of free p-cresol: a prospective and cross-sectional analysis', *Clin Chem*. 2003 Mar; 49(3): 470–8. doi: 10.1373/49.3.470. PMID: 12600960

Wikoff WR, Anfora AT, Liu J, Schultz PG, Lesley SA, Peters EC, Siuzdak G. 'Metabolomics analysis reveals large effects of gut microflora on mammalian blood metabolites', *Proc Natl Acad Sci USA*. 2009; 106(10): 3698–703

Nicholson JK, Holmes E, Kinross J, Burcelin R, Gibson G, Jia W, Pettersson S. 'Host-gut microbiota metabolic interactions', *Science*. 2012; 336(6086): 1262–7

Org E, Blum Y, Kasela S, Mehrabian M, Kuusisto J, Kangas AJ, Soininen P, Wang Z, Ala-Korpela M, Hazen SL, Laakso M, Lusis AJ. 'Relationships between gut microbiota, plasma metabolites, and metabolic syndrome traits in the METSIM cohort', *Genome Biol*. 2017; 18(1): 70

Does testosterone have balls when it comes to ageing?
Morley JE, Haren MT, Kim MJ, Kevorkian R, Perry HM 3rd. 'Testosterone, aging and quality of life', *Journal of Endocrinological Investigation*. 2005; 28(3 Suppl): 76–80. PMID: 16042363

Min KJ, Lee CK, Park HN. 'The lifespan of Korean eunuchs', *Curr Biol*. 2012 Sep 25; 22(18): R792–3. doi: 10.1016/j.cub.2012.06.036. PMID: 23017989

Brown-Borg HM. 'Hormonal regulation of longevity in mammals', *Ageing Res Rev*. 2007 May; 6(1): 28–45. doi: 10.1016/j.arr.2007.

02.005. Epub 2007 Feb 20. PMID: 17360245; PMCID: PMC1978093

Schooling CM, Zhao JV. 'Investigating the association of testosterone with survival in men and women using a Mendelian randomization study in the UK Biobank', *Sci Rep*. 2021 July 7; 11(1): 14039. doi: 10.1038/s41598-021-93360-z. PMID: 34234209; PMCID: PMC8263740

Schooling CM, Au Yeung SL, Freeman G, Cowling BJ. 'The effect of statins on testosterone in men and women, a systematic review and meta-analysis of randomized controlled trials', *BMC Med*. 2013; 11: 57

Sievers C, Klotsche J, Pieper L, Schneider HJ, März W, Wittchen HU, Stalla GK, Mantzoros C. 'Low testosterone levels predict all-cause mortality and cardiovascular events in women: a prospective cohort study in German primary care patients', *Eur J Endocrinol*. 2010 Oct; 163(4): 699–708. doi: 10.1530/EJE-10-0307. Epub 2010 Aug 4. PMID: 20685832

Araujo AB, Dixon JM, Suarez EA, Murad MH, Guey LT, Wittert GA. 'Clinical review: Endogenous testosterone and mortality in men: a systematic review and meta-analysis', *J Clin Endocrinol Metab*. 2011 Oct; 96(10): 3007–19. doi: 10.1210/jc.2011-1137. Epub 2011 Aug 3. PMID: 21816776; PMCID: PMC3200249

Dunn M, Mulrooney KJ, Forlini C, van de Ven K, Underwood M. 'The pharmaceuticalisation of "healthy" ageing: Testosterone enhancement for longevity', *Int J Drug Policy*. 2021 Sep; 95: 103159. doi: 10.1016/j.drugpo.2021.103159. Epub 2021 Feb 12. PMID: 33583680

Alexander SE, Pollock AC, Lamon S. 'The effect of sex hormones on skeletal muscle adaptation in females', *Eur J Sport Sci*. 2021 May 18: 1–11. doi: 10.1080/17461391.2021.1921854. Epub ahead of print. PMID: 33890831

Alexander SE, Abbott G, Aisbett B, Wadley GD, Hnatiuk JA, Lamon S. 'Total testosterone is not associated with lean mass or handgrip strength in pre-menopausal females', *Scientific Reports*. 2021; volume 11, pp. 1–9. doi: 10.1038/s41598-021-89232-1

Morrison D, Hughes J, Della Gatta PA, Mason S, Lamon S, Russell AP, Wadley GD. 'Vitamin C and E supplementation prevents some of the cellular adaptations to endurance-training in humans', *Free Radical Biology and Medicine*. 2015; volume 89, pp. 852–862. doi: 10.1016/j.freeradbiomed.2015.10.412

And what about oestrogen?

Strong R, Miller RA, Antebi A, Astle CM, Bogue M, Denzel MS, Fernandez E, Flurkey K, Hamilton KL, Lamming DW, Javors MA, de Magalhães JP, Martinez PA, McCord JM, Miller BF, Müller M, Nelson JF, Ndukum J, Rainger GE, Richardson A, Sabatini DM, Salmon AB, Simpkins JW, Steegenga WT, Nadon NL, Harrison DE. 'Longer lifespan in male mice treated with a weakly estrogenic agonist, an antioxidant, an α-glucosidase inhibitor or a Nrf2-inducer', *Aging Cell*. 2016 Oct; 15(5): 872–84. doi: 10.1111/acel.12496. Epub 2016 Jun 16. PMID: 27312235; PMCID: PMC5013015

Mishra SR, Chung HF, Waller M, Mishra GD. 'Duration of estrogen exposure during reproductive years, age at menarche and age at menopause, and risk of cardiovascular disease events, all-cause and cardiovascular mortality: a systematic review and meta-analysis', *BJOG*. 2021 Apr; 128(5): 809–821. doi: 10.1111/1471-0528.16524. Epub 2020 Nov 5. PMID: 32965759

Lacreuse A, Mong JA, Hara Y. 'Neurocognitive effects of estrogens across the adult lifespan in nonhuman primates: State of knowledge and new perspectives', *Horm Behav*. 2015 Aug; 74: 157–66. doi: 10.1016/j.yhbeh.2015.03.001. Epub 2015 Mar 8. PMID: 25762288

Garratt M, Leander D, Pifer K, Bower B, Herrera JJ, Day SM, Fiehn O, Brooks SV, Miller RA. '17-α estradiol ameliorates age-associated sarcopenia and improves late-life physical function in male mice but not in females or castrated males', *Aging Cell*. 2019 Apr; 18(2): e12920. doi: 10.1111/acel.12920. Epub 2019 Feb 10. PMID: 30740872; PMCID: PMC6413653

Garratt M. 'Why do sexes differ in lifespan extension? Sex-specific pathways of aging and underlying mechanisms for dimorphic responses', *Nutrition and Healthy Aging.* 2020; 5: 247–259. doi: 10.3233/NHA-190067

Tezil T, Chamoli M, Ng CP, et al. 'Lifespan-increasing drug nordihydroguaiaretic acid inhibits p300 and activates autophagy', *npj Aging Mech Dis.* 2019; 5: 7. https://doi.org/10.1038/s41514-019-0037-7

Harrison DE, Strong R, Alavez S, Astle CM, DiGiovanni J, Fernandez E, Flurkey K, Garratt M, Gelfond JAL, Javors MA, Levi M, Lithgow GJ, Macchiarini F, Nelson JF, Sukoff Rizzo SJ, Slaga TJ, Stearns T, Wilkinson JE, Miller RA. 'Acarbose improves health and lifespan in aging HET3 mice', *Aging Cell.* 2019 Apr; 18(2): e12898. doi: 10.1111/acel.12898. Epub 2019 Jan 27. PMID: 30688027; PMCID: PMC6413665

Antibiotics – living longer, living shorter

Houtkooper R, Mouchiroud L, Ryu D, et al. 'Mitonuclear protein imbalance as a conserved longevity mechanism', *Nature.* 2013; 497: 451–457. https://doi.org/10.1038/nature12188

Hutchings MI, Truman AW, Wilkinson B. 'Antibiotics: past, present and future', *Curr Opin Microbiol.* 2019 Oct; 51: 72–80. doi: 10.1016/j.mib.2019.10.008. Epub 2019 Nov 13. PMID: 31733401

Lynn MA, Eden G, Ryan FJ, Bensalem J, Wang X, Blake SJ, Choo JM, Chern YT, Sribnaia A, James J, Benson SC, Sandeman L, Xie J, Hassiotis S, Sun EW, Martin AM, Keller MD, Keating DJ, Sargeant TJ, Proud CG, Wesselingh SL, Rogers GB, Lynn DJ. 'The composition of the gut microbiota following early-life antibiotic exposure affects host health and longevity in later life', *Cell Rep.* 2021 Aug 24; 36(8): 109564. doi: 10.1016/j.celrep.2021.109564. PMID: 34433065

Antioxidant supplements

Myung SK, Ju W, Cho B, Oh SW, Park SM, Koo BK, Park BJ; Korean Meta-Analysis Study Group. 'Efficacy of vitamin and antioxidant supplements in prevention of cardiovascular disease: systematic review and meta-analysis of randomised controlled trials', *BMJ.*

2013 Jan 18; 346: f10. doi: 10.1136/bmj.f10. PMID: 23335472; PMCID: PMC3548618

Jenkins DJA, Kitts D, Giovannucci EL, Sahye-Pudaruth S, Paquette M, Blanco Mejia S, Patel D, Kavanagh M, Tsirakis T, Kendall CWC, Pichika SC, Sievenpiper JL. 'Selenium, antioxidants, cardiovascular disease, and all-cause mortality: a systematic review and meta-analysis of randomized controlled trials', *Am J Clin Nutr.* 2020 Dec 10; 112(6): 1642–1652. doi: 10.1093/ajcn/nqaa245. PMID: 33053149; PMCID: PMC7727482

Forman, H.J., Zhang, H. 'Targeting oxidative stress in disease: promise and limitations of antioxidant therapy', *Nat Rev Drug Discov.* 2021; 20: 689–709. https://doi.org/10.1038/s41573-021-00233-1

Part 6 – It's not so bad to change what's on the outside

Bonell S, Murphy SC, Griffiths S. 'Under the knife: Unfavorable perceptions of women who seek plastic surgery', *PLoS One.* 2021 Sep 7; 16(9): e0257145. doi: 10.1371/journal.pone.0257145. PMID: 34492078; PMCID: PMC8423238

Brooks AT. 'Aesthetic anti-ageing surgery and technology: women's friend or foe?', *Sociol Health Illn.* 2010 Feb 1; 32(2): 238–57. doi: 10.1111/j.1467-9566.2009.01224.x. Epub 2010 Feb 8. PMID: 20149147

Garnham B. 'Designing "older" rather than denying ageing: problematizing anti-ageing discourse in relation to cosmetic surgery undertaken by older people', *J Aging Stud.* 2013 Jan; 27(1): 38–46. doi: 10.1016/j.jaging.2012.11.001. Epub 2012 Nov 21. PMID: 23273555

Garnham B. 'A cutting critique: Transforming "older" through cosmetic surgery', *Ageing and Society.* 2014; 34(8): 1356–1379. doi:10.1017/S0144686X1300010X

Roh DS, Panayi AC, Bhasin S, Orgill DP, Sinha I. 'Implications of Aging in Plastic Surgery', *Plast Reconstr Surg Glob Open.* 2019 Jan 14; 7(1): e2085. doi: 10.1097/GOX.0000000000002085. PMID: 30859042; PMCID: PMC6382222

'Patients must come first: regulate cosmetic surgeons like any other doctor', *Sydney Morning Herald*, 2021 Nov 1. https://www.smh.com.au/national/patients-must-come-first-regulate-cosmetic-surgeons-like-any-other-doctor-20211031-p594qb.html

Ricciardelli R, White P. 'Modifying the Body: Canadian Men's Perspectives on Appearance and Cosmetic Surgery', *The Qualitative Report*. 2011; 16(4): 949–970. https://doi.org/10.46743/2160-3715/2011.1115

Part 7 – While you're waiting on the magic pill of youth

Palmore EB. 'Predictors of the longevity difference: a 25-year follow-up', *Gerontologist*. 1982 Dec; 22(6): 513–8. doi: 10.1093/geront/22.6.513. PMID: 7152310

Gellert C, Schöttker B, Brenner H. 'Smoking and All-Cause Mortality in Older People: Systematic Review and Meta-analysis', *Arch Intern Med*. 2012; 172(11): 837–844. doi:10.1001/archinternmed.2012.1397

Arima H, Barzi F, Chalmers J. 'Mortality patterns in hypertension', *J Hypertens*. 2011 Dec; 29 Suppl 1: S3–7. doi: 10.1097/01.hjh.0000410246.59221.b1. PMID: 22157565

Willadsen TG, Bebe A, Køster-Rasmussen R, Jarbøl DE, Guassora AD, Waldorff FB, Reventlow S, Olivarius Nde F. 'The role of diseases, risk factors and symptoms in the definition of multimorbidity – a systematic review', *Scand J Prim Health Care*. 2016 Jun; 34(2): 112–21. doi: 10.3109/02813432.2016.1153242. Epub 2016 Mar 8. PMID: 26954365; PMCID: PMC4977932

Turner, E.L., Dobson, J.E. & Pocock, S.J. 'Categorisation of continuous risk factors in epidemiological publications: a survey of current practice', *Epidemiol Perspect Innov*. 2010; 7, 9. https://doi.org/10.1186/1742-5573-7-9

Hydes T, Buchanan R, Kennedy OJ, Fraser S, Parkes J, Roderick P. 'Systematic review of the impact of non-alcoholic fatty liver disease on mortality and adverse clinical outcomes for individuals with chronic kidney disease', *BMJ Open*. 2020 Sep 28;

10(9): e040970. doi: 10.1136/bmjopen-2020-040970. PMID: 32988952; PMCID: PMC7523199

Hou, W., Yu, X., Fan, X. et al. 'The association of 14-year dietary cholesterol trajectories with the risk of cardio-metabolic diseases, all-cause mortality and serum lipids', *Eur J Clin Nutr.* 2021; 75, 283–290. https://doi.org/10.1038/s41430-020-00825-x

Part 8 – Does the mind matter?

Tran-Duy A, Smerdon DC, Clarke PM. 'Longevity of outstanding sporting achievers: Mind versus muscle', *PLoS One.* 2018 May 3; 13(5): e0196938. doi: 10.1371/journal.pone.0196938. PMID: 29723296; PMCID: PMC5933783

Garatachea N, Santos-Lozano A, Sanchis-Gomar F, Fiuza-Luces C, Pareja-Galeano H, Emanuele E, Lucia A. 'Elite athletes live longer than the general population: a meta-analysis', *Mayo Clin Proc.* 2014 Sep; 89(9): 1195–200. doi: 10.1016/j.mayocp.2014.06.004. Epub 2014 Aug 12. PMID: 25128074

Zhang M, Lv X, Chen Y, Tu L, Fan Z, Yao Y, Yu X, Guan N, Wang H. 'Excessive sleep increased the risk of incidence of cognitive impairment among older Chinese adults: a cohort study based on the Chinese Longitudinal Healthy Longevity Survey (CLHLS)', *Int Psychogeriatr.* 2021 Mar 4: 1–10. doi: 10.1017/ S1041610221000168. Epub ahead of print. PMID: 33658084

Brandts L, van Tilburg TG, Bosma H, Huisman M, van den Brandt PA. 'Loneliness in Later Life and Reaching Longevity: Findings from the Longitudinal Aging Study Amsterdam', *J Gerontol B Psychol Sci Soc Sci.* 2021 Jan 18; 76(2): 415–424. doi: 10.1093/ geronb/gbaa145. PMID: 32880641; PMCID: PMC7813181

Lee LO, James P, Zevon ES, Kim ES, Trudel-Fitzgerald C, Spiro A, III, Grodstein F, Kubzansky LD. 'Optimism is associated with exceptional longevity in 2 epidemiologic cohorts of men and women', *Proceedings of the National Academy of Sciences of the United States of America.* 2019; 116(37): 18357–18362. doi:10.1073/pnas.1900712116

Gutman D, Rivkin E, Fadida A, Sharvit L, Hermush V, Rubin E, Kirshner D, Sabin I, Dwolatzky T, Atzmon G. 'Exceptionally Long-Lived Individuals (ELLI) Demonstrate Slower Aging Rate Calculated by DNA Methylation Clocks as Possible Modulators for Healthy Longevity', *Int J Mol Sci.* 2020 Jan 17; 21(2): 615. doi: 10.3390/ijms21020615. PMID: 31963520; PMCID: PMC7013521

Fastame MC, Penna MP, Hitchcott PK. 'Psychological markers of longevity in Sardinian centenarians: the impact of developmental factors and social desirability', *Aging Clin Exp Res.* 2020 Jan; 32(1): 107–114. doi: 10.1007/s40520-019-01157-y. Epub 2019 Mar 13. PMID: 30868424

Fastame MC, Mulas I, Pau M. 'Mental health and motor efficiency of older adults living in the Sardinia's Blue Zone: a follow-up study', *Int Psychogeriatr.* 2020 Sep 1: 1–12. doi: 10.1017/S1041610220001659. Epub ahead of print. PMID: 32867876

Dunlop K, Victoria LW, Downar J, Gunning FM, Liston C. 'Accelerated brain aging predicts impulsivity and symptom severity in depression', *Neuropsychopharmacology.* 2021 Apr; 46(5): 911–919. doi: 10.1038/s41386-021-00967-x. Epub 2021 Jan 25. PMID: 33495545; PMCID: PMC8115107

Christman S, Bermudez C, Hao L, Landman BA, Boyd B, Albert K, Woodward N, Shokouhi S, Vega J, Andrews P, Taylor WD. 'Accelerated brain aging predicts impaired cognitive performance and greater disability in geriatric but not midlife adult depression', *Transl Psychiatry.* 2020 Sep 18; 10(1): 317. doi: 10.1038/s41398-020-01004-z. PMID: 32948749; PMCID: PMC7501280

Ridout KK, Ridout SJ, Price LH, Sen S, Tyrka AR. 'Depression and telomere length: a meta-analysis', *J Affect Disord.* 2016; 191: 237–247

Brown PJ, Wall MM, Chen C, Levine ME, Yaffe K, Roose SP, Rutherford BR. 'Biological Age, Not Chronological Age, Is Associated with Late-Life Depression', *J Gerontol A Biol Sci Med Sci.* 2018 Sep 11; 73(10): 1370–1376. doi: 10.1093/gerona/glx162. PMID: 28958059; PMCID: PMC6132120

Nenadic I, Dietzek M, Langbein K, Sauer H, Gaser C. 'BrainAGE
    score indicates accelerated brain aging in schizophrenia, but not
    bipolar disorder', *Psychiatry Res Neuroimaging.* 2017; 266: 86–89
Fuller-Rowell TE, Homandberg LK, Curtis DS, Tsenkova VK,
    Williams DR, Ryff CD. 'Disparities in insulin resistance between
    black and white adults in the United States: The role of lifespan
    stress exposure', *Psychoneuroendocrinology.* 2019 Sep; 107: 1–8.
    doi: 10.1016/j.psyneuen.2019.04.020. Epub 2019 Apr 29. PMID:
    31055182; PMCID: PMC6635018
Shalev I, Entringer S, Wadhwa PD, Wolkowitz OM, Puterman E, Lin
    J, Epel ES. 'Stress and telomere biology: a lifespan perspective',
    Psychoneuroendocrinology. 2013 Sep; 38(9): 1835–42. doi:
    10.1016/j.psyneuen.2013.03.010. Epub 2013 Apr 29. PMID:
    23639252; PMCID: PMC3735679
Schiele MA, Gottschalk MG, Domschke K. 'The applied
    implications of epigenetics in anxiety, affective and stress-
    related disorders – A review and synthesis on psychosocial
    stress, psychotherapy and prevention', *Clin Psychol Rev.* 2020
    Apr; 77: 101830. doi: 10.1016/j.cpr.2020.101830. Epub 2020 Feb
    4. PMID: 32163803
Zhang T, Yan LL, Chen HS, Jin HY, Wu C. 'Association between
    allostatic load and mortality among Chinese older adults: the
    Chinese Longitudinal Health and Longevity Study', *BMJ Open.*
    2021 Aug 3; 11(8): e045369. doi: 10.1136/bmjopen-2020-045369.
    PMID: 34344673; PMCID: PMC8336121
Robertson T, Beveridge G, Bromley C. 'Allostatic load as a predictor of
    all-cause and cause-specific mortality in the general population:
    Evidence from the Scottish Health Survey', *PLoS One.* 2017 Aug
    16; 12(8): e0183297. doi: 10.1371/journal.pone.0183297. PMID:
    28813505; PMCID: PMC5559080
McEwen BS, Gianaros PJ. 'Central role of the brain in stress and
    adaptation: links to socioeconomic status, health, and disease',
    Ann N Y Acad Sci. 2010; 1186: 190–222. PMID: 20201874
Cohen S, Janicki-Deverts D. 'Can We Improve Our Physical Health
    by Altering Our Social Networks?', *Perspect Psychol Sci.* 2009

July; 4(4): 375–8. doi: 10.1111/j.1745-6924.2009.01141.x. PMID: 20161087; PMCID: PMC2744289

Fratiglioni L, Paillard-Borg S, Winblad B. 'An active and socially integrated lifestyle in late life might protect against dementia', *Lancet Neurol.* 2004 June; 3(6): 343–53. doi: 10.1016/S1474-4422(04)00767-7. PMID: 15157849

Stephens MA, Wand G. 'Stress and the HPA axis: role of glucocorticoids in alcohol dependence', *Alcohol Res.* 2012; 34(4): 468–83. PMID: 23584113; PMCID: PMC3860380

Jopp DS, Park MKS, Lehrfeld J, et al. 'Physical, cognitive, social and mental health in near-centenarians and centenarians living in New York City: findings from the Fordham Centenarian Study', *BMC Geriatr.* 2016; 16: 1. https://doi.org/10.1186/s12877-015-0167-0

https://www.abc.net.au/radionational/programs/healthreport/young-people-poorly-served-by-young-peoples-mental-health-servic/13631362

Firth J, Siddiqi N, Koyanagi A, Siskind D, Rosenbaum S, Galletly C, Allan S, Caneo C, Carney R, Carvalho AF, Chatterton ML, Correll CU, Curtis J, Gaughran F, Heald A, Hoare E, Jackson SE, Kisely S, Lovell K, Maj M, McGorry PD, Mihalopoulos C, Myles H, O'Donoghue B, Pillinger T, Sarris J, Schuch FB, Shiers D, Smith L, Solmi M, Suetani S, Taylor J, Teasdale SB, Thornicroft G, Torous J, Usherwood T, Vancampfort D, Veronese N, Ward PB, Yung AR, Killackey E, Stubbs B. 'The Lancet Psychiatry Commission: a blueprint for protecting physical health in people with mental illness', *Lancet Psychiatry.* 2019 Aug; 6(8): 675–712. doi: 10.1016/S2215-0366(19)30132-4. Epub 2019 Jul 16. PMID: 31324560

Schofield PE, Stockler MR, Zannino D, et al. 'Hope, optimism and survival in a randomised trial of chemotherapy for metastatic colorectal cancer', *Support Care Cancer.* 2016; 24: 401–408. https://doi.org/10.1007/s00520-015-2792-8

Schofield P, Ball D, Smith JG, Borland R, O'Brien P, Davis S, Olver I, Ryan G, Joseph D. 'Optimism and survival in lung carcinoma patients', *Cancer*. 2004 Mar 15; 100(6): 1276–82. doi: 10.1002/cncr.20076. PMID: 15022297

Goldilocks and sleep – What's 'just right' for living long?

Trudel-Fitzgerald C, Zhou E, Poole E, et al. 'Sleep and survival among women with breast cancer: 30 years of follow-up within the Nurses' Health Study', *Br J Cancer*. 2017; 116: 1239–1246. https://doi.org/10.1038/bjc.2017.85

Cappuccio FP, D'Elia L, Strazzullo P, Miller MA. 'Sleep duration and all-cause mortality: a systematic review and meta-analysis of prospective studies', *Sleep*. 2010 May; 33(5): 585–92. doi: 10.1093/sleep/33.5.585. PMID: 20469800; PMCID: PMC2864873

Shen X, Wu Y, Zhang D. 'Nighttime sleep duration, 24-hour sleep duration and risk of all-cause mortality among adults: a meta-analysis of prospective cohort studies', *Sci Rep*. 2016 Feb 22; 6: 21480. doi: 10.1038/srep21480. PMID: 26900147; PMCID: PMC4761879

Vaccaro A, Kaplan Dor Y, Nambara K, Pollina EA, Lin C, Greenberg ME, Rogulja D. 'Sleep Loss Can Cause Death through Accumulation of Reactive Oxygen Species in the Gut', *Cell*. 2020 Jun 11; 181(6): 1307–1328.e15. doi: 10.1016/j.cell.2020.04.049. Epub 2020 Jun 4. PMID: 32502393

Kocevska D, Lysen TS, Dotinga A, et al. 'Sleep characteristics across the lifespan in 1.1 million people from the Netherlands, United Kingdom and United States: a systematic review and meta-analysis', *Nat Hum Behav*. 2021; 5: 113–122

Jonasdottir SS, Minor K, Lehmann S. 'Gender differences in nighttime sleep patterns and variability across the adult lifespan: a global-scale wearables study', *Sleep*. 2021 Feb; volume 44, issue 2, zsaa169. https://doi.org/10.1093/sleep/zsaa169

Fjell AM, Sørensen Ø, et al. 'Self-reported sleep relates to hippocampal atrophy across the adult lifespan: results from the Lifebrain consortium', *Sleep*. 2020 May; volume 43, issue 5, zsz280. https://doi.org/10.1093/sleep/zsz280

Knutson KL, von Schantz M. 'Associations between chronotype, morbidity and mortality in the UK Biobank cohort', *Chronobiol Int.* 2018 Aug; 35(8): 1045–1053. doi: 10.1080/07420528.2018.1454458. Epub 2018 Apr 11. PMID: 29642757; PMCID: PMC6119081

Keeping time – your body clocks and staying young

Gossan N, Boot-Handford R, Meng QJ. 'Ageing and osteoarthritis: a circadian rhythm connection', *Biogerontology.* 2015 Apr; 16(2): 209–19. doi: 10.1007/s10522-014-9522-3. Epub 2014 Jul 31. PMID: 25078075; PMCID: PMC4361727

Takahashi JS, Hong HK, Ko CH, McDearmon EL. 'The genetics of mammalian circadian order and disorder: implications for physiology and disease', *Nat Rev Genet.* 2008 Oct; 9(10): 764–75. doi: 10.1038/nrg2430. PMID: 18802415; PMCID: PMC3758473

Damiola F, Le Minh N, Preitner N, Kornmann B, Fleury-Olela F, Schibler U. 'Restricted feeding uncouples circadian oscillators in peripheral tissues from the central pacemaker in the suprachiasmatic nucleus', *Genes Dev.* 2000 Dec 1; 14(23): 2950–61. doi: 10.1101/gad.183500. PMID: 11114885; PMCID: PMC317100

Stokkan KA, Yamazaki S, Tei H, Sakaki Y, Menaker M. 'Entrainment of the circadian clock in the liver by feeding', *Science.* 2001 Jan 19; 291(5503): 490–3. doi: 10.1126/science.291.5503.490. PMID: 11161204

Balsalobre A, Brown SA, Marcacci L, Tronche F, Kellendonk C, Reichardt HM, Schütz G, Schibler U. 'Resetting of circadian time in peripheral tissues by glucocorticoid signaling', *Science.* 2000 Sep 29; 289(5488): 2344–7. doi: 10.1126/science.289.5488.2344. PMID: 11009419

Duncan MJ. 'Interacting influences of aging and Alzheimer's disease on circadian rhythms', *Eur J Neurosci.* 2020 Jan; 51(1): 310–325. doi: 10.1111/ejn.14358. Epub 2019 Feb 21. PMID: 30689226

Leng Y, Musiek ES, Hu K, Cappuccio FP, Yaffe K. 'Association between circadian rhythms and neurodegenerative diseases', *Lancet Neurol.* 2019 Mar; 18(3): 307–318. doi: 10.1016/S1474-4422(18)30461-7. Epub 2019 Feb 12. PMID: 30784558; PMCID: PMC6426656

Hood S, Amir S. 'The aging clock: circadian rhythms and later life', *J Clin Invest*. 2017 Feb 1; 127(2): 437–446. doi: 10.1172/JCI90328. Epub 2017 Feb 1. PMID: 28145903; PMCID: PMC5272178

Keeping your brain young

Kolbeinsson A, Filippi S, Panagakis Y, et al. 'Accelerated MRI-predicted brain ageing and its associations with cardiometabolic and brain disorders', *Sci Rep*. 2020; 10: 19940. https://doi.org/10.1038/s41598-020-76518-z

Moore K, Hughes CF, Ward M, Hoey L, McNulty H. 'Diet, nutrition and the ageing brain: current evidence and new directions', *Proc Nutr Soc*. 2018 May; 77(2): 152–163. doi: 10.1017/S0029665117004177. Epub 2018 Jan 10. PMID: 29316987

Diamond K, et al. 'Randomized Controlled Trial of a Healthy Brain Ageing Cognitive Training Program: Effects on Memory, Mood, and Sleep', *J Alzheimers Dis*. 2015 Jan 1; 1181–1191

Chen X, Liu Z, Sachdev PS, et al. 'Dietary Patterns and Cognitive Health in Older Adults: Findings from the Sydney Memory and Ageing Study', *J Nutr Health Aging*. 2021; 25: 255–262. https://doi.org/10.1007/s12603-020-1536-8

Gustavson DE, Panizzon MS, Kremen WS, et al. 'Genetic and Environmental Influences on Semantic Verbal Fluency Across Midlife and Later Life', *Behav Genet*. 2021; 51: 99–109. https://doi.org/10.1007/s10519-021-10048-w

Bahar-Fuchs A, Martyr A, Goh AMY, Sabates J, Clare L. 'Cognitive training for people with mild to moderate dementia', *Cochrane Database of Systematic Reviews*. 2019; issue 3. Art. no.: CD013069. doi: 10.1002/14651858.CD013069.pub2. Accessed 13 February 2022

Part 9 – Here's what you can do at any age

Here's what you can do if you're a parent or plan to become one

Tarry-Adkins JL, Ozanne SE. 'Nutrition in early life and age-associated diseases', *Ageing Res Rev*. 2017 Oct; 39: 96–105. doi: 10.1016/j.arr.2016.08.003. Epub 2016 Sep 1. PMID: 27594376

Here's what you can do if you're 50

Li Y, Schoufour J, Wang DD, Dhana K, Pan A, Liu X, Song M, Liu G, Shin HJ, Sun Q, Al-Shaar L, Wang M, Rimm EB, Hertzmark E, Stampfer MJ, Willett WC, Franco OH, Hu FB. 'Healthy lifestyle and life expectancy free of cancer, cardiovascular disease, and type 2 diabetes: prospective cohort study', *BMJ*. 2020 Jan 8; 368: l6669. doi: 10.1136/bmj.l6669. PMID: 31915124; PMCID: PMC7190036

The annual check-up and staying young . . .

Liss DT, Uchida T, Wilkes CL, Radakrishnan A, Linder JA. 'General Health Checks in Adult Primary Care: A Review', *JAMA*. 2021 June 8; 325(22): 2294–2306. doi: 10.1001/jama.2021.6524. PMID: 34100866

Part 10 – The air we breathe

Reyna MA, Bravo ME, López R, Nieblas EC, Nava ML. 'Relative risk of death from exposure to air pollutants: a short-term (2003–2007) study in Mexicali, Baja California, México', *Int J Environ Health Res*. 2012; 22(4): 370–86. doi: 10.1080/09603123.2011.650153. Epub 2012 Mar 15. PMID: 22420489

Rajagopalan S, Landrigan PJ. 'Pollution and the Heart', *N Engl J Med*. 2021 Nov 11; 385(20): 1881–1892. doi: 10.1056/NEJMra2030281. PMID: 34758254

Landrigan PJ, Fuller R, Acosta NJR, et al. 'The Lancet commission on pollution and health', *Lancet*. 2018; 391: 462–512

Pope CA 3rd. 'Respiratory disease associated with community air pollution and a steel mill, Utah Valley', *Am J Public Health*. 1989 May; 79(5): 623–8. doi: 10.2105/ajph.79.5.623. PMID: 2495741; PMCID: PMC1349506

Dockery DW, Pope CA 3rd, Xu X, Spengler JD, Ware JH, Fay ME, Ferris BG Jr, Speizer FE. 'An association between air pollution and mortality in six U.S. cities', *N Engl J Med*. 1993 Dec 9; 329(24): 1753–9. doi: 10.1056/NEJM199312093292401. PMID: 8179653

Krewski D, Jerrett M, Burnett RT, Ma R, Hughes E, Shi Y, Turner MC, Pope CA 3rd, Thurston G, Calle EE, Thun MJ, Beckerman

B, DeLuca P, Finkelstein N, Ito K, Moore DK, Newbold KB, Ramsay T, Ross Z, Shin H, Tempalski B. 'Extended follow-up and spatial analysis of the American Cancer Society study linking particulate air pollution and mortality', *Res Rep Health Eff Inst.* 2009 May; (140): 5–114; discussion 115-36. PMID: 19627030

Brunekreef B, Beelen R, Hoek G, Schouten L, Bausch-Goldbohm S, Fischer P, Armstrong B, Hughes E, Jerrett M, van den Brandt P. 'Effects of long-term exposure to traffic-related air pollution on respiratory and cardiovascular mortality in the Netherlands: the NLCS-AIR study', *Res Rep Health Eff Inst.* 2009 Mar; (139): 5–71; discussion 73–89. PMID: 19554969

https://www.iarc.who.int/wp-content/uploads/2018/07/pr221_E.pdf

End note: Climate change, environmental stress, the abuse of medicine and living shorter

https://www.ipcc.ch/report/ar6/wg1/downloads/report/IPCC_AR6_WGI_SPM_final.pdf

https://www.ipcc.ch/report/ar5/wg2/human-health-impacts-adaptation-and-co-benefits/

Allison DB, Fontaine KR, Manson JE, Stevens J, VanItallie TB. 'Annual deaths attributable to obesity in the United States', *JAMA.* 1999 Oct 27; 282(16): 1530–8

Adair T, Lopez AD, 'The role of overweight and obesity in adverse cardiovascular disease mortality trends: an analysis of multiple cause of death data from Australia and the USA', *BMC Med.* 2020; 18: 199. https://doi.org/10.1186/s12916-020-01666-y

Preston SH, Mehta NK, Stokes A. 'Modeling obesity histories in cohort analyses of health and mortality', *Epidemiology.* 2013 Jan; 24(1): 158–66. doi: 10.1097/EDE.0b013e3182770217. PMID: 23211348; PMCID: PMC3870658

Rentería E, Jha P, Forman D, Soerjomataram I. 'The impact of cigarette smoking on life expectancy between 1980 and 2010: a global perspective', *Tob Control.* 2016 Sep; 25(5): 551–7. doi: 10.1136/tobaccocontrol-2015-052265. Epub 2015 Aug 25. PMID: 26307052

Index

rifampicin 106
  rapamycin, combined with
    106
risk factors
  multiple risk factor reduction
    178
  predictive tools 178–9
risk perception 199–200
Rothko, Mark 85
running 127, 130

salt 180–2, 215
  effects of 180, 181
  heart disease 180
  RDI 181
  sodium 181
sanitation 11
sarcopaenia 68, 71, 81
Sardinian people 200
saturated fats 82, 140
schizophrenia 31, 201
  brain age gap (BAG) 201
  life expectancy gap 201
screen time 211, 214, 219
Seeger, Pete 56
selenium 150
self-harm 22, 54, 200
Semmelweis, Dr Ignaz 11
senescent cells 44, 61, 118–21,
    125
  ageing and 120, 121
  causes 119, 122
  exercise and 126, 127
  healthy response, when 120
  secretions by 120, 127

senolytics 117, 120
  anti-ageing drugs, as 121
  human clinical trials 121
  potential, list of 121
sexual activity 176–7
  unsafe sex 177
short chain fatty acids (SCFAs)
    138, 140, 141
Silver, Dr Margery 15
sirolimus see rapamycin
    (sirolimus)
SIRT1 enzyme 91
  resveratrol and 91–3
skin cancer 36
sleep
  chronotype, individual 205
  circadian rhythms 72–3,
    204–5, 210
  dementia and poor sleep 206
  disrupted patterns 206
  insomnia 209
  light and 212, 214
  long 203, 204, 207, 208, 209
  night owls 205–6
  quality 209
  recommended range 208
  screens, light from 211, 214,
    219
  short 203, 204, 207
  sleep hygiene 210
  sleep restriction therapy 210
  sleep therapies 209–10
  sleeping pills 210
  studies, limitations of 204,
    208